MW00764687

Also by Jennifer Brush

Environment and Communication Assessment Toolkit for Dementia Care

A Therapy Technique for Improving Memory: Spaced Retrieval

Jennifer Brush & Kerry Mills

I Care

A Handbook for Care Partners of People with Dementia

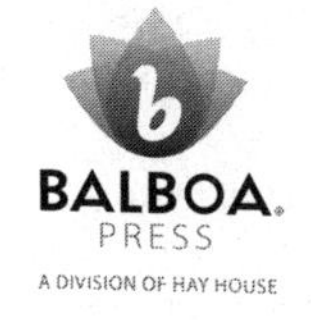

Copyright © 2014 Jennifer Brush & Kerry Mills.

All rights reserved. No part of this book may be used or reproduced by any means, graphic, electronic, or mechanical, including photocopying, recording, taping or by any information storage retrieval system without the written permission of the publisher except in the case of brief quotations embodied in critical articles and reviews.

Balboa Press books may be ordered through booksellers or by contacting:

Balboa Press
A Division of Hay House
1663 Liberty Drive
Bloomington, IN 47403
www.balboapress.com
1 (877) 407-4847

Because of the dynamic nature of the Internet, any web addresses or links contained in this book may have changed since publication and may no longer be valid. The views expressed in this work are solely those of the author and do not necessarily reflect the views of the publisher, and the publisher hereby disclaims any responsibility for them.

The author of this book does not dispense medical advice or prescribe the use of any technique as a form of treatment for physical, emotional, or medical problems without the advice of a physician, either directly or indirectly. The intent of the author is only to offer information of a general nature to help you in your quest for emotional and spiritual well-being. In the event you use any of the information in this book for yourself, which is your constitutional right, the author and the publisher assume no responsibility for your actions.

Printed in the United States of America.

ISBN: 978-1-4525-9073-8 (sc)
ISBN: 978-1-4525-9074-5 (e)

Library of Congress Control Number: 2014901470

Balboa Press rev. date: 05/29/2014

To my mom and dad—thank you.
Your love, guidance, and encouragement have
been the foundation to all that I am.
—Cookie Tunes

To E.B., the light of my life
To A.B., the love of my life
—J.B.

Contents

Appendix

Thank You

Our whole-hearted thanks to all of the people with dementia and their families who have made this book possible. Thank you for inviting us into your homes and your lives, for teaching us and for trusting us, and for sharing your stories, struggles, and victories.

Thank you to Barb Schmitz, Catherine Mills, and Chris Day for your editorial guidance and encouragement.

We extend our deep gratitude to George, Joanne, Charlie, Katie, Marv, Elfriede, Charlotte, and Jack for your contributions to furthering the goal of this book, which is to be an aid to every care partner.

Preface

To my family and friends,

I want to say thank you. I don't always say it, and I am not even aware of how often I should say it, but again thank you. If my mind was clear and I could access all the words in my heart, I would still struggle to express my gratitude.

I am most grateful for the love you have shown to me, especially when I make it difficult. Thank you for letting me do things and engage in my own life, even though it might cause more work for you at times. Thank you for not reminding me how much work I am causing you. Your encouragement is uplifting.

Thank you for not pointing out everything I do wrong and instead recognizing that I sometimes work so hard to do the simplest things. I appreciate that you value my effort more importantly than my outcome.

Thank you for always including me, talking to me, and not treating me like I am sick. I am so aware of what goes on around me, and your effort to keep me involved makes the world of difference to me each day.

While I don't know what tomorrow holds, or how I will act, or what I will say, thank you for treating me like the person I have worked toward being my whole life. Thank you for respecting me and for being so patient with me.

I know it is not easy for you all the time, but I do hope that I have provided some relief, some joy, and some laughs for you along the way. I hate to think I am the only one receiving. I thank you for being my partner.

Love,
Your loved one with dementia

Introduction

Our hope in writing this book for you and your loved one with dementia is to have a fulfilling, loving, and nurturing relationship and to minimize any depression and stress you might feel when caring for someone you love. Every chapter has many useful and practical suggestions to help you feel empowered, rather than defeated, while dealing with the daily trials of dementia.

I Care will help you change how you think about dementia. If you change how you think about the condition, you will change your approach. Your attitude toward dementia and toward your loved one will have a huge impact on your perception and how the disease will affect your life.

Through years of experience working with people with Alzheimer's disease and related dementias, we have learned what is necessary to prepare for the future while living in the present, how to make the most of your day, where to look for help when you need it, how to communicate effectively with someone with memory loss, and where to make changes in your home so it is safe. *I Care* clearly explains the essential information you need to be the best care partner you can be. As you gain more understanding regarding the unique needs of someone with dementia and initiate the strategies we suggest, your overall stress will lessen and your sense of being overwhelmed will diminish.

Although Alzheimer's disease and other forms of dementia present daily challenges, we have confidence that this book will help you focus on the joys of what still is, rather than what is not. Despite the despair that many families speak of, we believe there is more to the story and therefore want to offer you hope. There will be days (hopefully many) when you will laugh; there will be days when you will be surprised by your own strength; there will be days when you learn new things about the person you have known for most of your life; there will be days when you realize your great love for this person; and there will be days when you will be acutely aware of his or her great love for you.

Despite how your relationship with dementia started, you now have the opportunity to enjoy what might arguably be some of your best days yet and some of the best days for your loved one as well!

Chapter I

Controlling Yourself, Not the Circumstances

Reading this book is a good first step toward getting the help and support we all need to face the challenges of dementia. Because of the physiological changes in the brain that cause symptoms of dementia, we are incapable of changing the person with dementia. But we can help the person succeed, function independently, and live a full life. We can do this by changing our own behaviors. This will bring about substantial change in our journey through this disease process. It is important to recognize that the first change required will be within you.

When someone helps care for someone else, we call him or her a caregiver. This is a natural title and one we all understand; however, when we use this title to identify a person who provides care to a person with dementia, we are missing an important part of the relationship, as this "title" implies that there is nothing left for the person with dementia to contribute. By referring to "care partners," we are recognizing their contribution as "partners." With whom are they partners? They are partners *with* the person who has dementia. This means that they are not only giving but also receiving—the same as the person with dementia. This is the first step toward changing your perspective. This also means you, the care partner, need to prepare yourself to receive as well.

The following is a touching and enlightened account of how our friend Charles Farrell became a care partner.

> *My wife Carol, now seventy-seven years old, has been fearful of dementia for most of her adult life. Her mother was diagnosed with Alzheimer's disease at sixty-seven when Carol was in her late thirties. After several attempts of failed home care, Carol's mom was placed in a nursing home, where she remained for eight years until her death. Our early experience with institutional care was very disheartening, so we decided that if either of us ever faced the possibility of needing long-term care, we would make every effort to care for each other in our own home.*
>
> *We were in our early forties when Carol's mom died. Although our possibility of needing long-term care seemed very remote, we began to adjust our lifestyle with the aim of remaining physically fit and healthy.*
>
> *Our first encounter with the possibility of dementia moving into our lives occurred approximately eight years ago when Carol underwent a neurological evaluation for an unrelated health problem. During Carol's discussion with the neurologist, she brought up her fear of Alzheimer's disease. Given the fact that she noticed some difficulty remembering familiar recipes and following directions, she asked if there was any possibility that she might be developing Alzheimer's disease. The physician suggested that memory problems such as these were common in our age group and that this did not necessarily indicate the presence of the disease.*
>
> *Carol was then scheduled to have an MRI of her brain to rule out any structural problems. We were*

told that the scan would be helpful in discovering anatomical evidence of Alzheimer's disease. After completing the scan, the neurological examination, and numerous other tests, we were told that Carol had no signs of Alzheimer's disease. Carol remained concerned and asked if there were any other tests that might be done to further evaluate her risk for the disease. The physician recommended that she undergo a neuropsychological examination. After multiple interviews, we were told that Carol demonstrated some evidence of declined executive function. She eventually received a diagnosis of MCI (mild cognitive impairment), a symptom complex that leads to Alzheimer's disease in 85 percent of cases. Approximately three years later, Carol was diagnosed with Lewy body dementia. At this point, we reaffirmed our commitment to care for each other and to do so in our own home.

Being a retired surgeon, I had always considered myself to be a "caregiver." To me, that meant being in charge of any situation that might occur. I promptly hired a contractor and told Carol that we needed to remodel and create a bedroom and bath on the first floor. That was perfectly obvious to me, but it was not so obvious to Carol. The next year or so was very difficult. It took me a long time to realize that although I was trying to be a "caregiver," I was, in fact, stripping Carol of control of her life.

Carol had now begun to move into the "world of dementia," and I was denying her perception of reality. I was trying to make her accept my view of reality and, in the process, was destroying her persona. She just couldn't understand! Duh! She really was unable to understand. I needed to learn to become a care partner and not just a caregiver. I needed to move into the world of dementia with her and see things through her eyes, to accept and validate her reality. It is not my job to change her. It is my job to change our environment so that we can live in it together.

To become a care partner, one first has to be present. This is far different from just being there. I needed to focus intently on Carol—her needs and her wishes. Morrie, Carol's little Cavalier King Charles spaniel, is by far her best care partner. Morrie is always present. He sits by her side, and his big, brown eyes seem to be focused on nothing but Carol. More importantly, Morrie can read Carol's mind. In Morrie's nonverbal world, he knows when Carol is anxious and moves closer. He sits by her side or on her lap, if possible. When she is calm, he sits quietly and watches. He perceives her needs and says yes to her every wish.

In the world of dementia, nonverbal communication is critical. Every move is a form of communication, as is every grimace and every smile. If Carol becomes anxious and acts out, or attempts to strike someone, she is not becoming "violent" because she has Alzheimer's disease. She is frustrated and upset because something in her environment is causing her grief. It is our job to determine what it is and to make the environment comfortable for her.

Carol can no longer string words together and form sentences. She frequently says, "Go home." I have learned that she does not want to leave the room that she knows is her home, but there is something in the room that does not feel like home to her. During one of these episodes, we took a trip around the room in her wheelchair, and I noticed that she stared angrily at her favorite blue chair. The chair was facing the TV set and not next to the end table. Once I moved the chair to where it "belonged," Carol was "home."

Carol's Alzheimer's has not stolen all of her memory nor destroyed who she is. Even though it has made it more difficult for her to string her remaining memories together, she is still here. It is up to us—me, our little "village" of family, and friends—to find her. We have enjoyed tremendous support from this group. Our youngest daughter, along with her husband and son, lived with us during the early years of our journey. Family meals occur on a weekly basis, and friends drop in regularly to share a meal and camaraderie. The grandkids share their holidays, birthdays, graduations, and most of their special events.

Social groups that Carol was a part of over the years, such as the Church Chicks and the Knit Wits, all make regular visits. We are welcomed to social events sponsored by a local running group, with which we have been associated for more than thirty years. Our Unitarian Universalist Church welcomes Carol with open arms and big smiles when we arrive for Sunday services. Carol's very special friend, with whom she worked at high school fundraisers many years ago, has shared morning exercise and breakfast three to four days a week for the last eight years.

We are not alone! We remain a vibrant part of our little village, which we love very much and which continues to love and support us. This group shines a bright light on our family and brings us out of the shadows and fog of dementia.

My youngest daughter, the Reverend Katie Norris, and I cofounded The Carolyn L. Farrell Foundation for Brain Health, whose mission is to empower those affected by dementia and mental illness through art care and community outreach. This allows us to serve the greater community in which we live and provides me with a long-term goal.

In the past two years, we have moved into the magical, mystical, intimate, silent world of dementia. This is truly a wonderful place. Our home has become quiet. At night, it is essentially silent. I sleep in a small bed next to Carol, and frequently we awaken at the same time. I care for her physical needs in silence. We then move close together. I place my arm around her shoulder and my head on her chest and feel totally relaxed. I feel her breath as I count her respirations and feel her heart beat. If Carol is anxious and fearful, our vital bodily functions are out of sync. As we simply lie together, we become closer and closer together and finally, truly, become one. We are as much in love today as we have ever been in the last fifty-plus years.

Dementia has not robbed Carol of her personality, and it has not robbed us of each other. We have simply become partners.

Work on Managing, Not Controlling

The key is effective management, not control. It's a natural tendency for the care partner to try to control the environment and every situation that occurs in much the same way that a parent controls every aspect of an infant's life. The needs of an infant are few and relatively simple, and the life experience is almost nonexistent. You cannot use the same approach, or anything like it, when caring for a senior adult with dementia because his or her needs are much more varied and complex, and life experience is almost at full capacity. The person with dementia has led a full life and remembers many of his or her jobs and experiences. A person with dementia should not be treated as a child since he or she is an adult.

A completely new mindset is required in order to effectively manage the environment and situations that arise as a result of dementia. Control is vital—but on the part of the care partner who must strive for a maximum degree of self-control. Only then will you have success in managing all things related to the person with dementia. Control connotes a takeover of someone's existence. Managing the person with dementia is a learned art that allows you to direct his or her natural abilities and choices to establish a balance of stability and harmony.

This mindset will require the care partner to practice self-discipline and create a constructive and proactive attitude by putting in place an infrastructure (groundwork) that generates the maximum degree of positive outcomes (possibilities) for the person diagnosed and the care partner. Here's how to get started.

Self-discipline

Melissa's mom lived a difficult life. She had a strict father and an abusive husband. She raised three children who loved her tremendously. Melissa and her siblings found a care home where their mom could walk freely and engage in many activities while her care and safety needs were met. Melissa would visit her mom a number of days a week and would join her mom in whatever activities she was doing. Every time she visited, Melissa had a huge smile on her face and brought joy to everyone who saw her, most importantly, to her mom.

Before or after her visit, Melissa would sometimes cry, thinking of what was happening to her mom; however, she never brought this sadness

> *to her mom. Many family friends would speak with Melissa and ask about her mom. Melissa would tell them how she was doing and would discuss how she was changing with the disease's progression. These friends would often comment, "It will be good when she is not suffering anymore." Melissa would become very defensive to these types of comments and say, "Mom has it so good now. She is loved, and no one is hurting her. This is the happiest I have ever seen her, and I want her to have this as long as possible."*

Having self-discipline is about controlling yourself, not about controlling others. Becoming self-disciplined is hard work and requires practice. So often, care partners try to control the situation by attempting to control the person with dementia. For instance, if a person with dementia is rummaging through the closet, we tell the person to "stop rummaging" or "sit at the table." If he or she does not comply, the care partner becomes frustrated. If this happens more than a few times, the care partner will often lose his or her patience. In this situation, the care partner needs to control his or her response and give the person with dementia something that is "acceptable" to rummage through or invite the person to do something else that he or she is interested in doing.

Often, care partners will direct the person with dementia because they feel they have to control what the person is doing. However, when this backfires and the person with dementia resists the control, care partners become exhausted. This results in frustration for both the care partner and the person with dementia, and things usually escalate from there. Offering the person with dementia choices, instead of telling him or her what to do often works better than providing constant direction. Instead of trying to control the person, now is the time to begin looking at how you can control yourself to minimize arguments, upsetting conversations, and anger.

Attitude

Jessica's mother was a fairly absent parent when Jessica was growing up. She wasn't around to put her on the school bus, didn't show up at school plays, and wasn't even around on most holidays. Jessica longed to have a relationship with her mom in which she felt loved, accepted, or at the least, acknowledged. Her mother lived a life of fame and put her own interests before those of anyone else.

When her mother was diagnosed with dementia after having a stroke, Jessica responded the way any "loved" daughter would have and hopped into the driver's seat to care for her mom. Her mom continued to resent her and the things Jessica was doing for her. Jessica's attitude toward her mom was quite astounding; she loved her mom because she was her mother, not because of how her mom treated her. As she cared for her mother throughout the years of her decline, their relationship began to change.

After her mom passed away, Jessica wrote the following as a reflection of her life with her mother during the disease. "You would be pleased to know that I was with her for her last hours, and it was a very profound experience filled with much love, forgiveness, caring and true connection as mother and daughter. I saw her take her last breath and felt privileged to be with her right up to the last moment. It was the greatest gift I could give her—to be of comfort in her last hours and minutes. In

> *retrospect, one can see how everything happens as it should, and if the opportunities are recognized and taken advantage of to the highest purpose, even suffering and misfortune can be turned into blessings. This is how I have come to view the journey my mother and I had traveled together, ending in a place of incredible peace and love."*

Jessica chose to give herself the gift of forgiveness. It was an opportunity for her to stop judging her mother. It offered her peace. Living with dementia is not easy, and caring for someone with dementia is often harder; no disease is easy to live through. No misfortune, no illness, no loss is ever welcomed. It is not usually pleasant, and yet, so many people will talk of the good that came out of a negative situation. Simultaneously, there are just as many people who complain about their situations and say nothing good can come out of them. Here is a positive opportunity to take control. What do you choose to see? Which experience do you choose to have? Which path will you choose? You have the choice about what attitude you will bring to this situation.

> *Attitude is everything, so pick a good one.*

If you change how you think about this disease, you will change how you approach it. Your attitude toward this disease and toward your loved one with the disease will have a huge impact on your perception and how the disease will affect your life.

Take a minute to examine your attitude. Are you angry? Are you sad? Are you asking, "Why us?" All of these questions are normal, expected, and perfectly natural. However, are you angry with your loved one because he or she has dementia? If so, then now is a good time to reevaluate your attitude toward him or her. A person with dementia is a person. This person is observant, hears well (barring a hearing problem), sees well (again, barring vision conditions), knows how you treat him or her, recognizes your tone of voice, picks up on nonverbal communication, and to some degree, does all these things better than most of us.

That being the case, it is best to treat him or her like a person. Being angry or upset with your loved one isn't going to make the person feel better or act differently. In most cases, the person will respond to this negativity by becoming apathetic, or worse, defensive. This behavior will only serve to agitate you and provoke your loved one into being angry and upset. Always keep in mind that this person is dealing with a disease. He or she is living life with a disease that is causing the brain to physically malfunction, to operate while it is broken, and to complete a puzzle, if you will, with missing pieces. The person is aware that things aren't right, but he or she doesn't always realize his or her contribution to the problem.

Joe and Karen, his care partner, went to the park and had an ice cream. It was a great day. Joe leaned over to Karen and whispered, "I just wanted to tell you that I am losing my mind." A person with dementia is aware that something is wrong. However, the fear, uncertainty, and embarrassment of saying something can often make the person resist talking about it. If you, as the care partner, are approachable, non-argumentative, and do not show disappointment, the person with dementia will be more likely to talk to you. Your attitude will dictate so much of what this disease looks like for your loved one. This is a huge responsibility and not one to take lightly. We do not suggest this to add pressure to your role, but to remove the pressure. Do your best to have fun, slow down, and enjoy the simple moments.

Groundwork

> *As part of Julie's job, she used to visit one particular care home on a monthly basis. This home she visited was about two hours from her house. Upon her arrival, she would spend some time visiting with the residents.*
>
> *One day, she met a lady named Ruth and they began chatting. Just as Julie turned to leave the room, Ruth raised her voice and said, "You are a beautiful girl." Julie beamed and felt good about what she had chosen to wear that day. However, before she took another step, Ruth added, "And you know, dear, I am legally blind!"*

Who we are is not always evident, and what we bring to the table is not always visible, but who we are often brings out certain reactions in others, and our contributions are most obvious in how others respond to us. Because of this, it is imperative that our interactions with people diagnosed with dementia are deliberate and consistent.

After learning that a loved one has been diagnosed with Alzheimer's or one of the several related dementias, most people don't know where to turn. Do you join a support group? Do you spend hours scouring the Internet to learn more about it? Do you call all your family and tell them? Do you lock yourself in your room and cry? The truth is that you might do all of these things or you might do none of these things; everyone reacts differently. However, what will allow you to stay one step ahead of this disease is to prepare the groundwork and create a foundation that will support you, the care partner, as well as the person diagnosed.

In order to make interactions with your loved one as rewarding as possible for you both, it is essential that you adopt a mindset of preparedness. This includes:

Leaving your frustration, sadness, and anger in the bathroom, outside, on the golf course, etc.

Reflect on things that make you smile to improve your happiness quotient. Write some of them here:

1) ______________________
2) ______________________
3) ______________________

Have a ready supply of things you can share with your loved one at your fingertips. Good examples are jokes, Dear Abby's, animal stories, the weather, local town news, and pictures of grandchildren. It is easy to collect these from the Internet and e-mail.

Give up the need to be right. As a person progresses in the disease, he or she will struggle with many things, including memory, sense of time, numbers. For instance, when a person with dementia recounts a story, it often differs from the care partner's account. There is nothing gained by trying to correct the person with dementia. He or she will probably not remember anyway, which will cause you further frustration. Don't strive to win the argument; strive to create harmony!

Show affection. Hold hands and give the person a hug. In many of our relationships, when we get frustrated or annoyed by someone, we often withhold affection. We wait until we calm down and feel better before we hug or kiss the person. In many of these situations, however, showing affection reminds both parties that there is still mutual love, which can help diminish negative emotions.

Laugh often. We really mean this. If you have nothing to laugh about, break out your old photo albums and take a walk down memory lane. Watch a comedian or invite your grandchildren over to play. Find something that makes you laugh, and incorporate this into your regular routine.

When people visit, always include the person with dementia in the conversation. For instance, if your son comes to visit and asks how Dad is doing, encourage him to direct the question to his father. If a waiter asks you what your husband would like to order, look at him and ask him if he is in the mood for his favorite meal. It is a wonderful thing to know that people love us and want to care for us, but most people still prefer to care for themselves and enjoy their independence.

Exercise together. Whether it's going for a walk each day or doing a yoga class together, carve out time to exercise. What is good for the body is good for the brain. Avoid telling your loved one that he or she needs to exercise. Instead, ask him or her to join you because you need it.

Decide what you would like to do each day, and then make it happen. It's best to plan thirty-to-sixty-minute activities that won't be derailed easily by interruptions.

Possibilities

Maggie, an only child, was in her late thirties when her mother, Rose, was diagnosed with Alzheimer's disease. This was especially hard for Maggie because she lost her father to this same disease when she was only twenty-five years of age. Having just become the mother of twins when her mother was diagnosed, she had no choice but to find a home to care for her mom. Maggie suffered from a lot of guilt because she felt she should have cared for her mom at home, the way her mom had cared for her dad. Maggie would visit several times a week and was a vocal advocate for her mom.

During the time her mom was living in this care home, the activity director began teaching Rose how to use Skype (video teleconferencing). At first, Rose was very confused. When she would hear Maggie's voice, Rose would walk around the room and look for her daughter. Over the course of a few months, Rose was able to focus on the computer screen and say "hello" before getting up and leaving. Her attention span was very limited.

On the evening of Maggie's thirty-seventh birthday, the director and Rose Skyped her and sang "Happy Birthday." As soon as they finished, Rose got up and walked away.

Maggie sat at the computer with tears in her eyes and said to the director, "You can't imagine how much I needed to hear my own mom wish me a happy birthday today."

One of the great heartaches that families experience is the sense of being forgotten by loved ones affected by dementia. For instance, people diagnosed with dementia soon begin to forget family birthdays, anniversaries, names, accomplishments, etc. However, if you provide some assistance and remind the person of these details, this person will typically respond in a manner he or she would have before the disease.

It is very easy to see what is missing, what is gone, and what is not right anymore. It is easy because this is where you, the care partner, are left to compensate. While this disease can have devastating effects on your loved one, it is important to adjust your expectations and find joy in the smaller, daily successes. This will help you, the care partner, to not be as overwhelmed, frustrated, and disappointed. By adjusting your expectations to be more reasonable and practical, your hard work and great effort will pay off, and you will experience greater satisfaction in your caregiving role.

By adjusting your expectations, you will be providing your loved one with more opportunities to succeed. So often, particularly in the later stages of the disease, families and professional care partners are quick to say that the person diagnosed is unable to speak, can't respond, etc. Often, however, if we kneel beside him or her and hold hands, the person will often turn to us, say hello, utter part of a sentence, or simply smile. It may be more efficient or practical for the care partner to limit communication with the person diagnosed, but this intervention only serves to diminish further the remaining capabilities of the loved one.

Webster's Dictionary defines *possible* as "being within the limits of ability, capacity, or realization." Within limits, a person with dementia is able to realize that his or her abilities are different than they used to be, which differs greatly from having no abilities. As families and care partners are able to identify what the person with dementia is really able to do, they are often surprised and encouraged to demonstrate more capabilities. Over time, the person with dementia grows more confident and is able to progress through the disease with a higher level of independence. He or she is less sad because you, the care partner, are helping the person adapt in a positive manner.

Many times, people will comment that these words of advice are easier said than done. We agree. Sometimes, they explain how the relationship was prior to the disease to reinforce how their loved one has diminished. Again, we understand. Nevertheless, our advice has merit and just requires either more self-discipline or a greater effort by the care partner. Ultimately, the loved one and the care partner will reap greater rewards for their efforts.

The average life span of a person with dementia is between eight and fifteen years. So we challenge you to make the most of these years for the sake of your loved as well as for yourself. There will not be a second act; there will not be an opportunity to relive these years. We encourage you to take time to recognize this reality along the way so you can live without regrets.

Chapter 2

Describing the Brain with Dementia

We must learn to appreciate and find joy in our loved ones instead of always seeking to change them. Build on a person's positive qualities and accept them for who they are.

Joe was a former New York City police officer. When he was twenty-four years old, he was working as a crossing guard and saw a really cute lady waiting to cross. He stopped traffic to let her cross, and as she passed, he thought she was really pretty. He watched where she went and when his break time came, he went to the restaurant where the lady had gone, and they started chatting.

Sixty years later, Joe retold this story of how he met his wife, every single morning to the ladies with whom he ate breakfast. The ladies would giggle as he talked about seeing Molly for the first time, and his eyes beamed as he took a picture of this beautiful redhead out of his wallet to show the ladies. No one tired of the story because they all had Alzheimer's disease. It was a wonderful way for everyone to start the day!

Imagine driving home from work and suddenly finding yourself on a street that does not look familiar. You search for a landmark—the corner gas station, the market where you buy milk, the drug store—but nothing is familiar. You begin to panic a bit until you see State Street. You think, *Good, I know I can take that road home.* When you get home, you say nothing to your spouse. It was a strange experience that you attribute to being tired.

The next day, you become very frustrated while trying to assemble a storage unit in the basement; you find the directions to be very confusing. A few days later, the bank sends you a letter that you bounced a check, and you receive an overdue notice for the electric bill that you are certain you paid. You sit down at the kitchen table to read the mail, drink a cup of coffee, and figure out what is going on.

Thirty seconds later, your spouse asks why you aren't dressed to go out to dinner. Going out to dinner is the furthest from your mind; you just wish that everyone would leave you alone so you had time to figure this out!

We have all been lost, encountered nonsensical directions, and forgotten to pay a bill or two. For someone with dementia, however, these problems occur gradually, become more frequent, and then persist. It's frustrating to have trouble doing something you have always done without a problem. It's scary to feel like your world is falling apart or that you are losing your mind. A person with dementia knows that there is something wrong and struggles to make it right. Dementia causes changes within the brain over which the person has no control.

This chapter provides a brief overview of how the brain works and what happens when it is damaged. We have been told over and over that as people understand what is happening in the brain, it is so much easier to be patient and understanding in the care partnering role. Furthermore, we then focus on how to embrace these changes to maintain a harmonious relationship. We in no way mean to replace seeking information from a physician or reading a comprehensive medical guide about dementia. Rather, this section is written to give you a basic understanding of why you are observing certain changes in cognition, behavior, or language functioning in your loved one and what you can do to best support him or her.

Defining Dementia

Let's start with answering the question many people ask—what is the difference between dementia and Alzheimer's disease? Dementia is a symptom or a set of symptoms. It is not an actual disease, but a term used to describe a group of brain disorders that cause a loss in intellectual abilities, such as memory, language, visuospatial skills, calculation, abstract reasoning, judgment, and behavior. The changes are persistent and significant enough to interfere with daily life. Since dementia refers to a group of symptoms that accompany several diseases and conditions, it is very important to have a complete evaluation from your physician. See the appendix for questions to ask your physician.

There are several reversible or treatable causes of dementia. Some include:

- infections
- medication side effects
- vitamin deficiency
- depression
- severe hypothyroidism

Then there are the causes for dementia that are progressive and non-reversible. The most common causes of these dementias are:

- Alzheimer's disease
- vascular dementia
- frontal temporal dementia
- Parkinson's disease
- Lewy body dementia
- traumatic brain injury
- chronic alcohol or drug use
- depression
- brain tumors

Alzheimer's disease is the most common cause of dementia, and for this reason, the words dementia and Alzheimer's disease are often used interchangeably in conversation. The difference between the two is that dementia is a symptom, and Alzheimer's disease is a disease. Alzheimer's disease causes a person to exhibit symptoms of dementia. Listed above is a short list of the most common causes of dementia, which includes Alzheimer's disease.

Alzheimer's Disease

According to the Alzheimer's Association, approximately 5.4 million people are living with Alzheimer's disease in the United States. On a global scale, this number increases to 35.6 million. These numbers are growing at an alarming rate. By 2050, the Alzheimer's Association projects that 16 million Americans and 115.4 million people worldwide will have Alzheimer's disease. Just about everyone we know is touched by Alzheimer's disease in some way. We all have a friend, family member, neighbor, or colleague who is either living with the disease or helping care for someone who has the disease.

While the strategies discussed in *I Care* may not always be exactly applicable for all types of symptoms you are encountering, the interventions have been found to be very relevant and helpful for older adults who have a wide range of conditions that cause dementia.

The Brain 101

> Keep your brain healthy by exercising. Even a 30–40 minute walk three days a week will improve age-related loss of brain cells. So, get moving!

The brain is a very powerful and complex organ, which has the ability to affect the entire working of the body. So how does it work? In a short simple answer, it is a communication network, with neurons being the computers and phones, and the axons and dendrites being the wires and radio signals that allow them to share information. Neurons are specialized cells that make up our nervous system and transmit information from our brain to the rest of the body.

One neuron transmits an electrical signal (by way of the axon), which triggers the release of chemicals called neurotransmitters, to another neuron, which is received by the dendrites. The chemicals carry instructions that turn nearby brain cells on and off. This is how information is transferred through the brain. Scientists estimate that we have approximately 80–100 billion neurons in our brain.

To stay healthy, nerve cells must be able to communicate with each other, carry out metabolic activity, and repair themselves. Interrupted communications between neurons are the basis for the changes that we see in our loved ones. Alzheimer's disease is characterized by a loss or death of neurons, which causes atrophy of the brain. Scientists are still trying to determine the causes of these brain changes.

Memory

Common deficits related to Alzheimer's disease or other related forms of dementia that affect communication include memory lapses, impaired attention span, visual perceptual deficits, and hearing impairment. Communication impairments in people with Alzheimer's disease are largely explicable in terms of the disease's effect on memory. For example, people with Alzheimer's disease experience impairment in memory systems called episodic, semantic, lexical, and working memory, all of which can result in difficulty generating ideas, trouble maintaining a topic of conversation, and reduced vocabulary. A memory is actually a stored pattern created by the brain's neurons. Memory involves both the process of manipulating knowledge as well as the storing of knowledge. Although the ability to learn and recall information is impaired by Alzheimer's disease, not all aspects of memory and learning are equally affected.

Memory is not one thing, but a number of complex systems. As information enters through our five senses, it is encoded and then stored in our working memory. Working memory holds sensory information temporarily until it is either used at that moment or processed into long-term storage for later access.

There are two main forms of memory:

- *knowing how* (knowledge of skills)
- *knowing that* (knowledge of facts)

We commonly use the memory systems of the brain together. *Knowing that*, also referred to as declarative memory, is information that is retrieved consciously; people are aware that they are accessing the information.

One form of *knowing that* is episodic memory, or our autobiographical memory of the events of our life. Episodic memory stores information about the time and place when a particular event (or episode) occurred. You have probably spent time with a person with Alzheimer's disease or other related forms of dementia who asked the same question over and over. That is often, but not always, a result of a deficit in episodic memory. The person is not doing it on purpose; the person is seeking information that he or she cannot access or does not have stored in long-term memory. Let us say that again: the person is not doing this on purpose or to intentionally bother you.

In a case like this, it is very helpful to write down the answer to the person's question and put it on a bulletin board, dry-erase board, an index card, or someplace where it makes sense to encourage the person to look for information. If you practice reading the information with the person every time he or she asks the same question—instead of just telling the person the answer—over time, the person will develop the habit of going to that place to look for and read the information and will stop asking you (for more information, see "Practice at Remembering" in the "Staying Engaged" chapter).

Another kind of *knowing that* memory is semantic memory. This is a memory for facts or world knowledge and does not have to be linked to a particular event. Semantic memories are those that store general factual knowledge that is independent of personal experience. Examples include types of food, capital cities, and vocabulary. Because people with Alzheimer's disease or other related forms of dementia have difficulty accessing that memory of *knowing that*, they become disoriented to time, forget people's names, and cannot retain information in conversation, lose ideas about what to talk about, and repeat stories or questions.

Knowing how, or non-declarative memory, is memory that is reflected in how we do something; it's automatic. It is often called procedural memory. It includes motor and perceptual skills and habits. For example, when learning to play a musical instrument, you pay close attention and watch each hand position. As you practice and master the skill, it becomes part of your *knowing how* system. Later when you pick up your instrument, you are attentive to it, but your hands move automatically. It's just like riding a bike or reading. The skills become second nature and are easy to do. Other non-declarative skills include brushing teeth, cooking, playing board games, or participating in hobbies.

> While memory loss is a common symptom of dementia, memory loss by itself does not mean that a person has dementia.

Non-declarative memory is considered an area of preserved cognitive capability long through the course of Alzheimer's disease in particular. Because this memory system seems to be less impaired, non-declarative memory-based training has the potential of generating positive effects on functional change with this population. When we interact with a person with dementia, we want to do activities that use this memory system rather than putting an emphasis on possibly impaired episodic or semantic memory systems.

Attention

A person with Alzheimer's disease or other related forms of dementia also experiences changes in the ability to pay attention to things. Attention is the process of focusing on a specific stimulus for a particular length of time.

- *Selective attention* is the ability to focus on a single stimulus or process at one time while ignoring irrelevant or distracting information.
- *Sustained attention* is the ability to focus attention over extended periods of time.
- *Divided attention* is the ability to focus on more than one stimulus or process at one time or the ability to attend to multiple stimuli at the same time.

Research suggests that attention is the first non-memory area to be affected by Alzheimer's disease or other related forms of dementia, even before deficits in language or visuospatial functions (skills that enable us to visually perceive objects and the spatial relationships among objects).

Consider the person with Alzheimer's disease or other related forms of dementia who you know. What difficulties with daily tasks that might be related to attention deficits may have occurred in early stages? It appears that divided attention and aspects of selective attention are very vulnerable, while sustained attention is relatively preserved in the early stages of the disease. As a result, a person may be able to enjoy focusing on a jigsaw puzzle for an extended period of time in a quiet environment free from distractions, but an environment with significant amounts of noise, movement, or visual clutter will be over-stimulating and create difficulties locating a desired item, focusing on an activity, or remembering the sequence of tasks.

As a care partner, you'll need to look for things that may cause distractions and try to limit or avoid those situations. For example, if you are going out to dinner with friends, choose an early time before the restaurant is full and ask for a table that is away from noise and traffic patterns. This will help the person with dementia focus on the conversation. Creating cues or templates can also help a person focus, attend to, and complete a task. Think of a cue as a reminder, signal, or hint. Cues are part of the environment or material near the person that helps focus attention. Cues can be statements such as, "Take your medicine" or they can be symbols such as an X or an arrow pointing to where to begin reading.

Templates are guides that help someone complete a task. For example, a utensil tray in a drawer is a template. It has a cutout shape for each different piece of flatware, making it very clear where each piece should go. A common template used for a person with memory impairment is a placemat with an outline of the plate and each picture of a utensil printed on the placemat. This is something that can easily be made at home and covered with contact paper. This type of template shows the person that there is a place for everything and allows him or her to independently set the table without having to rely on memory skills. The point of using cues and templates is to allow the person to rely less on the *knowing that* memory and more on the *knowing how* memory.

Dysfunction of the Lobes

The brain is divided into two sections or hemispheres. Each cerebral hemisphere is divided into four lobes: the frontal, parietal, temporal, and occipital. Depending on the cause of dementia, different parts of the brain may be affected. With some diseases like Alzheimer's, eventually all parts of the brain are affected. If a person has a traumatic brain injury or a stroke, it is possible that only one part of the brain will be affected. Rather than trying to explain the progression of each disease, we have decided to explain how the different parts of the brain work so that as you see changes in your loved one, you will be able to see what is happening and what you can do to support the person.

Frontal Lobe

As the name suggests, the frontal lobes of the brain are located in the front. This lobe is responsible for higher-level cognitive functions, such as reasoning and judgment (called executive functions). People with executive dysfunction due to frontal lobe impairment generally do not know they have this dysfunction. Most importantly, the frontal lobe contains several cortical areas involved in the control of voluntary muscle movement, including those necessary for the production of speech and swallowing.

Impairment of the frontal lobe may result in the following:

- A lack of physical or verbal impulse control.

  - Socially inappropriate behavior, such as making rude comments or sexually inappropriate jokes. It is best to ignore this behavior and not pay it attention. We tend to react to this behavior, but doing so does not change the behavior. For some people, this lack of impulse control allows a person to be affectionate in a way that he or she may have never been. Many children have reported a loved one saying, "I love you," or hugging them when the loved one hadn't done that for most of his or her life.

  - Aggressive behavior, such as becoming easily angered while driving or pushing away a care partner during care because the person doesn't feel they need the help. You will only fuel the situation and make it worse by reacting to the behavior and expressing the same excitement. It is important to listen to what the person is saying and to stay calm when this happens. Giving the person space or just sitting with him or her quietly can often help the person calm down.

  - Less self-judgment. This allows a person with dementia to try new things without being self-critical. This explains why a person with dementia relates so well to different art projects and discussions. The person freely says whatever comes to mind!

- Difficulty thinking about multiple thoughts or multitasking.

  - When this first begins, it will be frustrating and seem like a great loss. As the dementia progresses, it can be viewed as a positive change because if the person is engaged in something enjoyable, he or she won't be focused on participating in other tasks, such as driving the car. So, if the person is engaged in something desirable, they won't be able to be doing something less preferable.

- Impairment of moral principle, hoarding, or shoplifting.

  - If shoplifting is a problem and you cannot leave the person at home while you are shopping, ask your loved one to push the cart or hold items for you so his or her hands are occupied. Try to engage the person by asking him or her to locate items on the shelf or to read the shopping list for you.

- Inability to do abstract reasoning, reduced ability for mathematical understanding.

  - The person may have trouble paying bills on time or balancing the checking account, but he or she may enjoy helping you by completing basic math problems or signing checks.

- Difficulty thinking of ideas for conversation or of possible explanations for an event.

  - When someone cannot remember why—or even if—a certain event occurred, the person's brain may try to "fill in the blanks." Your loved one may notice that there is a dent in the side of the car and report that someone ran into him or her, rather than realizing that he or she hit something.

- Difficulty recognizing when finished with a task or struggling to take the initiative to begin a task.
    - For individuals who were always self-starters, it is difficult for families to see this change. However, trouble getting started shouldn't be viewed as disinterest in doing things. If asked in a loving manner and given some assistance to get started, the person will regularly be ready to do anything!
- Lack of awareness for how much time has passed, impaired understanding of the sequence of events in past or present time.
    - Frequently, a person with dementia will become very anxious about appointments if told too far in advance. Because one's sense of time is impaired, the person may be anxious for days or hours beforehand. In this case, it is best to wait until very close to the appointment to tell the person.
- Difficulty adapting to new situations.
    - While damage to this part of the brain makes it more difficult for a person to adapt, it doesn't make a person incapable. You'll need to provide assurance and reminders along the way.
- Absence or disturbance of motion in a muscle, rigidity, or tremors

- Inform your physician if your loved one is experiencing these symptoms because an occupational or physical therapy evaluation may be warranted to determine the need for assistive devices to help with mobility, toileting, dressing, and grooming.

Temporal Lobe Impairment

The temporal lobes of the brain are essential for memory. The temporal lobes are also associated with auditory processing, the sense of smell, the ability to understand, and production of meaningful speech.

Impairment of the temporal lobe may result in the following:

- Struggle to understand conversation and directions.
    - Provide directions one step at a time and try writing them down on index cards. Show the cards to the person during the activity to improve comprehension. For example, write each step for getting dressed on a card in large print, and show the person the card while you help him or her carry out each step. Change the words on the card if necessary to make sure the person understands what it says. Pictures are also a great way to communicate steps.

- Difficulty producing the words one wants to use to communicate.
    - Be attentive to the person's gestures and body language. If the person has to struggle to find words, he or she may decide just to give up and stop trying. Be patient

and find ways to reduce the stress for the person. This may mean that you have to label commonly used items in the house so the person can just read the label when asking for things.

- Inability to remember what someone said five minutes prior.
    - Repetitive questioning is a common symptom of dementia. See the section about "Practice at Remembering" in the Staying Engaged chapter.
- Lack of understanding the meaning of words.
    - Pictures become very important when this happens. For example, you ask your care partner if he or she would like a grilled cheese sandwich, and your loved one says, "yes." When you bring this sandwich, the person says, "I don't want this." Our natural reaction is to respond in defense, "You just said you wanted it!" However, when someone processes language differently, we must realize that we can't depend on just words to communicate. In this case, you would be more successful to show a picture of the actual food.

Parietal Lobe Impairment

The parietal lobes have an important role in integrating our senses. The parietal lobe is associated with sensation, including the sense of touch, perception of warmth and cold, and of vibration. It is also involved in writing, some aspects of reading, as well as imagination and creativity.

Impairment of the parietal lobe may result in the following:

- Lack of recognition of objects or people in the environment.
    - Contrast helps people distinguish between different objects in the environment. It can also help draw the attention of people who have difficulty staying on task or establishing orientation. For instance, if a care partner is assisting a loved one with brushing his or her teeth and the toothbrush is the same color as the counter on which it rests, even if the care partner says, "Pick up the toothbrush," the person with dementia (not being able to see it easily) may not pick it up. Providing a toothbrush that contrasts in color with the counter might easily resolve this situation.
- Difficulty performing tasks that require manipulation of objects or of the body, such as getting dressed, washing dishes, or walking around objects or barriers.
    - Make sure there is a clear walking path through the rooms of the house. Remove clutter, cords, and throw rugs from the floor.
    - It is best to continue to keep individuals engaged in these activities to the degree one is able. A person might struggle to button a shirt, but can still zip a sweatshirt, or have difficulty tying shoes, but can manage Velcro shoes.
- Struggle to complete basic math problems or to write.

- Find tasks at which the person succeeds and use preserved abilities to complete those tasks successfully. For example, teaching a child a new song, telling a story about an event in one's childhood, or looking at pictures in a scrapbook.

- Responding to a request to walk or to move a part of one's body.

    - You may need to place your hand over your care partner's hand and provide physical assistance when beginning a task such as grooming or washing.

Occipital Lobe

The occipital lobes of the brain are mainly involved in processing information from the eyes. The ability to see objects is accomplished by the eyes, but the ability to make sense of what we see is the role of the occipital lobe. Sometimes damage of the occipital lobes can result in visual hallucinations or trouble with depth perception.

Impairment of the occipital lobe may result in the following:

- An inability to recognize objects. Often food, toilets, clothing, and other common daily objects are not perceived for what they are or for their intended purposes.

    - In this case, relying on written words to convey meaning may not be helpful. Routine, structure, and verbal cueing should be consistent to help your loved one be most successful.

- Trouble recognizing objects due to impaired depth perception.

    - For instance, a person might not eat potatoes if the plate is white because he or she can't see the white on white. It often happens that a person will wipe his or her mouth on a white tablecloth because they can't see the white napkin. If there is a red placemat in between the tablecloth and napkin, one will be more likely to use the napkin.

- Hallucinations can either be something they see that is not there at all or a misunderstanding of another object.

    - Hallucinations are common when a person has Lewy body dementia. It is best to respond to these hallucinations based on your loved one's reaction. In many cases, the hallucinations don't bother the person.

        - If the person tells you there are bugs all over, ask if the bugs are bothering him or her. If not, you do not need to respond to the hallucination. If the response is yes, ask where the bugs are so that you can dispose of them.

        - If the person is upset that "the man keeps coming over" you can tell the person you will lock the door so he can't come in. Disagreeing and telling him or her that there is not a man may cause the person to be afraid because he or she will feel that nothing can be done about it. By validating the person and doing something about the situation, he or she will be happy with you and feel more comfortable that someone is helping.

- If the person is not seeing an object for what it is (vision, shadows, and lighting all contribute to these hallucinations), you can label the object or remove it. If this is not an option, you can cover it and see if the person is less bothered by not seeing the object at all.

    - At dusk, be particularly mindful that objects outside can cause a person to react in what might seem to be a confused way. If the person is asking about things outside, make sure to look at it from the other person's perspective (his or her height, same lighting, etc.) to help you better understand what he or she is referring to.

As mentioned above, the changes in cognition and abilities occur as the lobe responsible for each function becomes damaged. The particular order and severity of each function varies with each individual person with dementia. When people we love experience changes in their brains, we have to make adjustments to our expectations. We begin to experience a "new normal" in our lives. This is what our friend Elfriede, a spouse and care partner, wrote to us about adjusting her expectations:

> *It was my birthday, the last one in my sixth decade and the first one without Fred in forty-two years. Fred was diagnosed with Alzheimer's disease over eight years ago, and he just went to live at a memory care home three months ago. It's been strange for both of us.*

Birthdays were always important celebrations in our family, and as I was driving myself to dinner with my brother and sister, I was reflecting on past birthdays. This year, all I wanted for my birthday was a kiss from my husband. Not much hope for that I supposed, but I made a small detour and stopped by to see Fred on my way to dinner. We sat on our usual bench, and I talked about my birthday while Fred listened. I reminisced about old times and told him my birthday wish was a little kiss. I talked some more and gave him a kiss on the check, saying it was time for me to go. With that, he very softly kissed my check and gave me all I could have asked for—a kiss and a smile in my heart. Strange how the world tilts, and a little kiss on a park bench is still one of the best gifts ever. Thank you, my darling, Elfriede.

Chapter 3

Putting Your Ducks in a Row

Living with dementia is a journey. Like all journeys, there will be an end. Live this journey without regret. Plan for tomorrow while you live for today.

Whether you are packing for a trip, preparing your kids for school, or making a shopping list, in most situations, being prepared makes everything go smoother. Although it is important to plan for the future and get your affairs in order, it is even more important to live in the present. It is fair to say that most people don't spend hours making a shopping list or packing for weeks for a simple weekend getaway. Being fully present in the emotional, physical, and mental aspects of our lives involves the self-control necessary to focus and engage with the world, while avoiding being distracted from what really matters. You must balance your time preparing for the future while you live for today. Preparedness is good, but all things in moderation.

When caring for a person with dementia, it is important to maintain that balance as well. Some people spend so much time trying to learn about the disease by reading every book or talking to all the people they know who have dealt with the disease. They explore every possible resource available in their areas; in doing so, they lose the time when their loved ones can best engage in relationships. Aside from not spending time with their loved one, care partners often spend so much time living the disease through other people's experiences that they are absent from their own lives. Being informed is important, but don't obsess about gathering information. You don't have to be an expert on dementia to be a good care partner.

In this chapter, we discuss practical, hands-on advice for how to prepare your attitude, perspective, home, and relationships. These preparations focus on minimizing emergencies and the hasty decisions that go along with them.

> *Fanny had two sons, Robert and Timmy. Fanny lived with Alzheimer's disease, and Timmy was diligent in making sure his mom was well cared for. We met this family after Fanny had already had the disease for a few years. Whenever Fanny was upset, I would talk about Timmy and she would smile; she was so proud of him. And of course, every time Timmy visited his mother, she would throw her arms up and wrap them around her son as she yelled out, "Timmy!" She would praise him and tell him how much she loved him!*
>
> *One day, about two years later, Timmy and I were talking and I mentioned how evident it was that his mom loved him. He shared with me that all his life, his mother never hugged him and never told him she loved him. He said, "I am not ready to lose my mom." Timmy went on to say that he truly believed that if his mother didn't have this disease, he never would have heard these three precious words and never would have experienced the affection of his loving mother.*

You can look at this situation as sad—sad that Timmy didn't have this love earlier in his life—or you can see the positive in this situation. As a grown man, Timmy received the long-awaited affirmation of his mother's love. Sometimes, it requires great trials in this life to enjoy the rewards that others so often take for granted. We can't emphasize enough that the first step to getting your ducks in a row is choosing a mindset to live in the moment. The rest of this chapter focuses on practical steps to ensure that you are prepared for the changes to come.

Legal Documents

Estate Planning

Estate planning is the process of anticipating and arranging for the disposal of your estate. It is important to plan ahead so that you can maximize the use and protection of your assets in case you have a dementia or another health problem in the future. You will have the satisfaction of knowing that your financial affairs are in order, and you won't leave a costly administrative nightmare to your loved ones.

When a person is diagnosed with any form of dementia, it is important to plan ahead financially so that you can maximize funds since health care costs increase over time. If you think you may need Medicaid services, find out about your state's eligibility requirements. You may need to get help from a financial planner or elder care lawyer as there are rules regarding spending your assets and regulations involving transferring those assets, which are imposed by various federal agencies. Considering that some events have implications even five years prior to a partner requiring care, professional advice should be sought as early as possible after a diagnosis.

Advance Directives

Advance directives are legal documents that allow you to state your preferences about end-of-life care ahead of time. It is important to have this conversation with a loved one who has been diagnosed so that you can execute his or her wishes. Some families suffer greatly because they do not know what their loved ones would have wanted and are overwhelmed by the responsibilities of making these decisions. If you discuss these things early, the family is left to follow their loved one's wishes. This discussion will help carry out this responsibility and can minimize guilt. We cannot stress enough how important this is!

Without these conversations and the proper documentation, families have been caught up in decisions being made for them that they have to undo, or worse yet, endure. Please don't delay; put these advance directives on your priority list. While it might be awkward and difficult to address these concerns, you can start by talking about what your wishes are and ask your loved one what they would like. This will make it less intimidating and scary for the person. We suggest that you meet with your lawyer or find a good eldercare lawyer in your area. Laws differ by state, and an eldercare lawyer will be able to inform you about your best options.

The most common forms of advance directives include:

- power of attorney
- health care proxy
- living will

A power of attorney document can appoint someone to take care of all of your affairs. This is called a general power of attorney. Or the power of attorney document can give a person the right to make only certain types of decisions, such as those related to health care or personal property. This is called a specific or limited power of attorney. You should choose someone that you trust to make good decisions on your behalf.

A health care proxy is a document that appoints someone to make medical decisions for you in the event that you become unconscious or incompetent. It is important to discuss your wishes ahead of time so that the proxy knows what you want.

A living will is a document that states which treatments you wish for if you are dying or permanently unconscious. You can designate any level or kind of medical care. This document will often include decisions regarding the use of artificial breathing machines or feeding tubes.

These documents are created together by an attorney to create a combination of legally empowered people and legal directions to them to ensure that the life decisions of the person with dementia are respected, and that they give legal control to people they choose.

Household Finances

In many cases, it is wise to transfer all finances and accounts related to bill paying into the name of someone other than the person with dementia. This includes credit cards, bank accounts, investment accounts, and other financial records. It is acceptable to keep a regular checking account with a small balance in this person's name to preserve a sense of empowerment for the person with dementia. As the person with dementia becomes more compromised, it can become a complicated legal mess to transfer the funds.

This is especially important for couples in which the person with dementia has always been the person responsible for bill paying. The spouse can always say, "I want to learn in case something should happen." It should never be phrased in such a way that the person with dementia "can't do it anymore." This is an opportunity for you, the spouse or loved one, to learn how.

While the person with dementia might be very possessive about this and become argumentative, it is important to reassure the person that you can still do the bookkeeping together. Assure the person that your goal is just to simplify things, not to take this away from him or her.

We recommend including the person in bill paying. Ask your loved one to write the checks, sign checks, put the bills in envelopes, etc. As his or her condition progresses and bill paying become overwhelming, it would be wise to minimize his or her involvement to only writing one check or signing one check. *It is important to ask the person if he or she would like to be included since they might be perfectly fine with relinquishing this responsibility. You will only know if you ask.*

Long-Term Care Insurance

If you have long-term care insurance, it is wise to contact the company before you need their services so you know what is required to activate services. Every policy is different, and it is best to become familiar with the insurance company when you are not in a time crunch or stressful situation. See the appendix for a list of questions to ask your insurance provider. Since you may need to reference the information in the future, it is prudent to document the answers.

Veterans Benefits

If the person with dementia is a veteran, contact your local Veterans Association (VA) to learn about benefits for which they are eligible. There are a great number of services available through this organization. It's best to call the VA directly and set up an appointment to find out how they can help.

Emergency Preparedness

The worst state to encounter is being unprepared in an emergency situation. Certain documents are important to have ready in an emergency. Prepare an emergency folder and keep it in a prominent place to which you have easy access. This folder should include the following information for the person with dementia:

- medical history
- current list of medications (include any medications used in the last two years that have been discontinued, and mark that they are not being given)
- any known allergies
- copy of health care proxy and power of attorney
- copy of insurance cards
- any preferred nicknames

- any known triggers that cause the person with dementia to become agitated
- any "quick tricks" to calm the person with dementia
- make sure to update this information whenever you go to the physician or the emergency room

Emergency Plan

If the spouse is caring for the person with dementia, it would be prudent to have the emergency folder for the spouse to minimize complications during the emergency. It is wise to put an emergency plan in place in the event something happens to the primary care partner.

- Use a medical alert system that allows you or your care partner to call for help if the person has fallen or is injured.

- If the spouse or primary care partner needs to leave the area to find help (or if going to the hospital for medical care), have a plan to ensure the safety of the person with dementia during the emergency.

- Decide who will be the first person called to join the person with dementia. This person should live close by. When this person is not available, decide who will be the second person called. Always be ready to call the back-up person.

- Be aware that the person with dementia may want to leave the home to find help. We recommend using a wander guard system to minimize the distance a person with dementia can go without anyone knowing. There are a number of everyday watches, bracelets, and shoes that have GPS devices in them that can be linked to a person's smartphone or be seen on the Internet. Many of them allow you to set an "invisible fence" so you are alerted when the person with dementia goes beyond these safe lines.

- For the person with dementia, keep a current list of daily activities, times, and the name and contact number of the person they do this activity with in a visible place. This will allow friends and family to help the person with dementia stick to a familiar routine during the time period after the emergency and before the spouse returns. The person with dementia will not necessarily be able to understand what is happening, and it will be best for the person to maintain his or her routine.

- For the person with dementia, keep a list of what medications she or he takes, the time they are taken, and where the medications can be found so the contact person can ensure your loved one continues to take them.

Many towns and counties have programs in which a person with dementia can be included in a registry that is accessible to local police, fire, and ambulance service personnel. Call your local police station and ask if they have a program in which you can register your loved one. This will help in the event your loved one wanders (common with almost a third of people diagnosed with dementia) and can be used to expedite services in the event of an emergency.

How to Be Most Prepared for a Physician's Appointment

The entire experience of physician appointments has changed tremendously over the last fifty years. Today's patient needs to be educated and prepared in order to give the physician tangible, relevant information to help the patient. See the appendix for suggested conversations to have with your loved one's physician. We consulted with geriatricians, physicians who are trained in working with the older population, while assembling this list.

The physician appointment scenario can be very stressful. Often, the reason a person with dementia needs to see the physician is because he or she has had some sort of change and/or are exhibiting an increase in anxiety, agitation, or other distress. As much as possible, document the concerns you have so that you can be clear when describing the situation to the physician. A person with dementia will often refuse to go to the physician, which makes the day of the appointment even more stressful. If you have questions and concerns already written down, you minimize the chance of leaving the physician's office without covering everything you wanted to discuss. Writing out your questions and ensuring you address all necessary issues will empower you and give you some control during this time. This will benefit you and your loved one.

In addition, if your loved one is exhibiting new symptoms, keep a log for one week so you (and other care partners, including the physicians) can clearly see what time of day the changes are happening and identify any triggers. Below is a sample log. See the appendix for a blank log.

Daily Log for (person with dementia):_____ Jordan_______
Dates: 8/6–8/12, 2013
Behavior that is being documented: ___________________
He is not sleeping at night___________________________

	Check if Sleeping	If awake, write if person is engaged, agitated, or has another behavior***
8:00 a.m.	X	
9:00 a.m.	X	
10:00 a.m.	X	
11:00 a.m.	X	
12:00 p.m.		Eats lunch (all of it)
1:00 p.m.		Goes for a walk
2:00 p.m.		Watches TV
3:00 p.m.		Watches TV
4:00 p.m.	X	
5:00 p.m.		Eats dinner (some of it)
6:00 p.m.		Watches TV
7:00 p.m.	X	
8:00 p.m.	X	
9:00 p.m.	X	
10:00 p.m.		Goes to the bathroom
11:00 p.m.	X	
12:00 a.m.		Goes to the bathroom
1:00 a.m.	X	
2:00 a.m.	X	
3:00 a.m.		Goes to the bathroom
4:00 a.m.		Walking around the house
5:00 a.m.		Walking around the house
6:00 a.m.		Tries to start getting ready for "work"
7:00 a.m.		Eats a bowl of cereal

The physician will rule out many conditions that might be causing the symptoms your loved one is experiencing and give you a hypothesis as to the cause. Many tests are required in order to obtain the most clear and accurate diagnosis of the specific cause for dementia symptoms. These usually include a physical exam, a medical history, blood tests, a neurological exam, cognitive testing, and brain imaging. Whenever possible, it is important to get a proper diagnosis. Many people wonder whether there is any value in going through this slew of tests to determine an actual cause of the disease. The reasons we feel there is merit for these tests include:

1. It is essential to rule out a person's cognitive impairment that is caused by a health condition that can be treated. For instance, a side effect of medication or an infection.
2. It is critical to pinpoint the specific type of dementia in order to optimize treatment when possible. Different diseases cause different symptoms of dementia. Knowing the specific cause greatly helps health care professionals develop proper treatment plans.
3. We don't know what the future holds in the way of medical treatment. In the event that there is a treatment option available that can help your loved one, you want to know as much information as possible while they are in the earlier stages of the disease.

However, if this series of testing causes your loved one with dementia great stress, then it is important to weigh the benefits versus the stress.

What About Medications?

People often ask us about specific medications for people with dementia. What helps, what doesn't, what should be taken, and what should not? While we are not physicians, we do suggest that a heart-to-heart conversation with your physician will give you an opportunity to learn more about available medications, side effects, and expected results. It is beneficial to share your feelings about medication—and what you are comfortable with—with your medical team. Often, families would like to see a loved one come off medications, but the doctor hesitates to do so when it is unclear how helpful the medication has been. Medical professionals don't want to remove any hope for how the medication might help; if the medication doesn't appear to be hurting the person with dementia, they may leave it in place.

In our experience, we suggest that families not depend solely on medication to resolve any symptoms they see in a loved one. If someone is agitated, we recommend assessing what might be causing this agitation so the triggers can be removed if possible. When someone is awake at night, try incorporating more exercise into the daily routine to help them sleep more naturally. If someone is resistant to trying new things, start by doing something that the person is comfortable with and then ask the person to try this new thing for a short time.

Lifestyle, level of physical activity, outlook on life, social networks, and family support all play significant roles in how successful someone is that experiences dementia and how successful you will be as a care partner. We don't discourage you from trying medication, but we do suggest that you do not depend solely on the medications to help with the needs of your loved one.

Your Direct Care Team

To start, recognize that you may not have to care for your loved one alone. However, you may need to pull your team together. Your care team might be composed of a spouse, children, siblings, grandchildren, friends, or nieces and nephews, all of whom have a different relationship with the person with dementia and are likely to have different ideas about what is best for the person. To some degree, you might all be correct. However, the most important and effective ingredient for the team members is to *work together* and keep the well-being of the person with dementia the *priority.* Due to lifelong relationship struggles and tensions, this might be very difficult for some families. In this case, the families can work with a third party to help them stay focused on how to best care for the person with dementia. A geriatric care manager is trained in doing just this. The stress of caring for someone with dementia is often overwhelming, and the stress of family arguments around caregiving must be minimized or preferably eliminated altogether.

Each friend and family member will react to the changes in the person with dementia differently. Sometimes, those who are most genuine and willing to help will not be able to help due to their own grief. While it will still be helpful to encourage them to stay involved, you, the care partner, might need to find someone else to fill their position. Likewise, some people who might be fearful or unavailable at first might become more comfortable as they become accustomed to the new role and may be more available as time goes on. No one should be judged during this time since each person processes the presence of the disease on his or her own. Judging people is a waste of energy on your part and further isolates them. Encourage people and make it easy for them to participate, but rely on those who are reliable—and don't worry about the others.

While many people may be willing to help, most people are uncomfortable if they don't know exactly what is expected of them. For this reason, it is helpful to give all people on the team a position. One person might have the position of making physician appointments and taking the person with dementia to the physician. Another person might have the position of scheduling a home care aide. Another person might have the position of ensuring that proper food is in the home. Someone else might have the position of power of attorney. These positions should also include responsibilities that generate fun and enjoyable activities. All care partners should carve out time for themselves to pay attention to and cultivate their own friendships and relationships. Strive to have a good balance.

Your family physician or primary care physician often will know the person with dementia best and be a great resource to the family. The family physician should notice and understand the changes your loved one is experiencing due to the long-time relationship. For situations in which the family physician is new, this relationship will be more for medical care and coordination of services. In either case, your primary care physician can advise you in assembling the rest of your dementia care team. Together, you can discuss including the following types of health care specialists on your team.

- Find a geriatrician and/or neurologist with experience in treating people with Alzheimer's disease and related dementias. A geriatrician specializes in health conditions related to aging, and a neurologist specializes in disorders of the nervous system, including the brain.

- Depression is common in people who have dementia. A psychiatrist, psychologist, or neuropsychologist is a mental health professional who can help you determine the type of treatment that will work best for your loved one.

- A geriatric nurse, social worker, or care coordinator can provide hands-on coordination and guidance in establishing a care plan that works for your family.

- A speech-language pathologist can help the person with dementia use strategies to preserve communication and cognitive functioning for as long as possible. If the individual has swallowing problems, the speech-language pathologist will work with the person to ensure safe swallowing. This may include teaching compensatory strategies or altering the person's diet so that he or she can eat without risk of choking or illness.

- An occupational therapist can provide help and training in undertaking daily activities, such as bathing, dressing, eating, playing, and participating in a favorite hobby. This professional will also assess and recommend equipment, such as mobility aids and wheelchairs, and suggest special devices to help around the home or workplace (if needed).

- It can be helpful to have someone come in to the home to help care for a person with dementia as the person's capabilities decline. As the primary care partner, you might want to call on a skilled nurse who is qualified in administering medications, as well as a home health care assistant who can help with bathing, dressing, or other daily routines.

Most people with dementia thrive when family and friends visit. Therefore, it is very effective for a person with dementia to perceive all care partners as friends rather than professionals. In order to accomplish this, care partners have to adopt a participative approach rather than a commanding approach. A commanding approach sounds like this, "It is time for you to eat" or "You have to take a shower." A participative approach sounds like this, "Would you like to eat with me?" or "Can I join you for breakfast?" or "Before we get started for the day, should we get freshened up?" Notice the participative approach will often end in a question, giving the person with dementia the opportunity to decide and giving him or her the control.

Louis led a very active life in his years of retirement. He volunteered at the local hospital, regularly worked out at the gym, and joined his friends for dinner a number of nights a week. When he started getting lost while driving, his family became very concerned. They anticipated a fight that they would surely lose. We discussed bringing in a home health aide to serve as a companion and driver and keeping him focused during his daily tasks.

Instead of having a long conversation about his overall state of cognition and asking him to stop driving (they already had that conversation), his family encouraged him to keep doing all he was doing and said they would like to give him the gift of a "chauffeur," to which he rolled his eyes. They

> *attempted to frame this gesture as simply a way of reducing stress for him and making his life easier.*
>
> *At first, Louis was very resistant, and a number of times, he left for his appointments before his chauffeur arrived. But after a few weeks, he began to make jokes about his chauffeur not wearing a black cap and began to enjoy his new buddy going to the gym with him and palling around with the guys. After a few months, Louis was no longer driving and found a new friendship.*

When a care partner interacts with a person with dementia doing social activities, they are often surprised by how much more successful the person can be. This perspective encourages the care partner to nurture the abilities still evident in the person with dementia. In addition, it provides a topic of conversation for the care partner and the person with dementia. Naturally, the hardest part is finding the right match for your loved one. See the appendix for interview questions and suggested answers when searching for the right care partner.

Different Types of Services

During the course of this disease, a person with dementia might engage with anywhere from one to ten different care services. These range from in-home care to a shared residential care setting. Therefore, we will spend a few minutes discussing the different options of care.

Personal Companions. These paid or unpaid staff members are companions or friends. A neighbor might fill this role, or you might hire someone through an agency or who works independently. This person should engage the person with dementia in things he or she likes to do. They should aim to have fun and be a source of stimulation for the person with dementia.

Home Health Aides. These paid staff serve the role of the companion (above) as well as providing personal care services. This staff is trained in providing hands-on personal care, such as bathing, dressing, and assistance in the bathroom. This staff can be hired through an agency or hired privately. It is important to make sure this care partner creates a relationship with the person with dementia and has good rapport with the primary care partner.

Social Model Day Programs. These are day programs that offer activities and snacks (sometimes meals) through the day. These are a great resource for people to engage with others in the same cognitive situation in an environment where they will not feel judged. Many people with dementia enjoy going (after a few weeks) and often make new friends. Encourage your loved one to try it for a few weeks and to not make a decision after the first day.

Medical Model Day Programs. These programs offer the same benefits of the social model day program but also concentrate on providing personal care, medications, and other medical needs. Since a person may need to qualify for this program, it is good to call ahead and ask what would be required.

Independent Senior Living. An apartment or small suite located in a larger building that provides basic services such as housekeeping, meals, and a concierge. Services will depend on the independent senior living center. Ask if they work with any specific home health aide agencies for when more services are needed. It is important to be up front with the staff of these residences so they can tell you if they are capable of providing for the needs of your loved one. Withholding information will only result in poor care for your loved one.

Assisted Living. This residence provides a higher level of support than independent senior living. They will generally offer a level of personal care that is included in the basic plans. This is more of a care home than an apartment. While residents have the freedom to come and go, there is usually a higher level of attention given to residents.

Memory Care Assisted Living. This residence provides a higher level of care than assisted living does. In most programs, there are fewer residents assigned to staff so that staff can help residents with all their needs. Often, the program space for memory care is secure so that residents cannot leave the care community unattended.

Nursing Home Care. This residence provides a higher level of care than memory care or assisted living communities do. They focus on medical needs. There is usually a nurse in the building twenty-four hours a day, and the number of residents that one staff cares for is higher than memory care assisted living.

Rehabilitation. This setting helps to care for patients who need rehabilitation services. These are usually short-term services after surgery, an acute illness, or broken bones. Depending on the level of care needed, a person can partake of rehabilitation services through home health care, as an outpatient at a rehabilitation clinic, or as an inpatient in a skilled nursing facility.

Palliative Care. This is intended to treat the discomfort of patients. This care is appropriate for people in all stages of a disease. There is no limit to how long a person might engage in this service. A person needs to qualify to receive services; in most states, a physician needs to sign the orders for a person to enroll in services.

Hospice Care. This is intended to make sure that people who are not expected to live more than a year are offered all services to make them comfortable. A person needs to qualify for these services; in most states, a physician needs to sign the orders for a person to enroll in these services. Oftentimes, families are scared of hospice because they see this as the end. However, for many families, hospice has provided an extra layer of support for families, extra attention to the person with dementia, and help in coordinating all areas of care. Many families report their mistake in calling too late because the service is often invaluable to families.

Preparing for a Move

Many families and people with dementia would like to stay in their own homes throughout the course of this disease. However, sometimes a move is inevitable for a person with dementia. There are a variety of reasons why a person with dementia may need to live in a shared residential setting. In this case, it is absolutely no reflection on you as a partner—you have not failed. Often, when families see their loved ones in this setting, they see that a team of professionals can provide a more comprehensive approach to care than a small family care team can.

The next question is usually, "When is the right time to move?" This is different for all families and depends on the size and involvement of care teams and how the person with dementia progresses. Families often wait until they are unable to care for the person at home any longer; however, there is nothing wrong with moving a loved one to a care center when the person is higher functioning when they can adjust better, manage change and transition, and make new friends. Any way you look at it, it is an important, yet difficult decision that must involve the person with dementia and the care team.

Here are some things to consider:

1. Plant the seed early. Find out about different programs in the community, and visit with your loved one. Discuss care options early, and find out about your care partner's preferences. Be honest about what you think you can do, and don't make any promises that you think you cannot keep. Every situation is different. Sometimes the best promise is to say, "Dad, I will always do the best thing for you." This will help eliminate guilt for you down the road and will reassure your loved one that you have his or her best interest at heart. *Never* threaten that if the person doesn't improve or do as you have asked that you will place the person in a home somewhere.
2. Expect a bit of nervousness or anxiety. Naturally, a move causes most people to be nervous because it's difficult to process how this change will affect all aspects of his or her life. It takes time to adjust to new surroundings. For a person with dementia, the issue of moving frequently causes anxiety and often refusal. One might respond by

saying, "I can't move. I have too much stuff," or "I won't know anyone," or "I am too old to move."

3. Address concerns honestly. It is important to address both verbalized concerns and nonverbal behaviors that may be indicting apprehension or worry. Assure the person that you will be able to visit often. Let your loved one know that he or she can bring personal belongings, will meet people with similar interests, and will make friends quickly, etc. Suggest a tour of the care community or a visit to meet the residents.
4. Remember, no decision is final. And there is no reason to tell your loved one anything different. If the person enjoys her/himself in a program, he or she should stay. If the person absolutely hates it, you should look to see what else there is in the local area that might be better suited to their needs. Make decisions one day at a time.

As you search for places to help you with long-term care in the United States, one resource you should explore is the Pioneer Network website (https://www.pioneernetwork.net). The Pioneer Network advocates for elders across the spectrum of living options and is working toward a culture of aging that supports the care of elders in settings where individual voices are heard and individual choices are respected, whether it is in nursing homes, transitional care settings, or wherever home may be.

We all feel that no one else will ever care for our loved ones the way that we do. In addition to this, there are unfortunately many residential care homes that accept people with dementia but evidently lack the understanding or resources to do so effectively. It is counterproductive for a family to fight with the facility or the staff. Working *with* the staff to see how they can best meet the needs of your loved one will be most advantageous. Rather than blaming the staff—the people who are doing their best to care for your loved one—ask them how you can help. Make the effort to ask a lot of questions, and share relevant information about your loved one with the staff.

The person with dementia is dealing with a degenerative disease. This means that they will continue to decline over time. In a setting that is not able to meet one's needs well, the person will be likely to decline more rapidly. If the care community cannot meet your needs, remember that you always have a choice. It is your job to be the advocate for yourself and your loved one.

Again, we can't emphasize enough that the first step to putting your ducks in a row is choosing a mindset to live in the present and cherish the moments. Don't spend your days waiting for tomorrow; look to see what your loved one is offering you today.

> *Thomas visited his great grandma, Nana Kitty, only a few times a year because they lived on opposite sides of the country. He was four years old when his Nana Kitty began experiencing severe short-term memory loss. His dad told him that Nana Kitty liked to play a game to see how many times in one visit she can say "I love you" and then hug Thomas.*
>
> *Thomas would run to his Nana Kitty and throw himself at her for hugs and then play and get up for hugs throughout his visit. He loved the game and thought his Nana Kitty was great at it. As he grew older, he became more aware that his Nana Kitty didn't remember things, but Thomas never said anything. Every time he would visit, he would play the game and love every minute. During one of his last visits with his Nana Kitty, he winked at his dad as he "played the game."*

Chapter 4

Staying Engaged

A relationship can be the very best thing that ever happened to us on one day—and the biggest source of frustration on another day. There can be a constant struggle between what our relationship really is and what we dream it can be. Throughout life, all the little things accumulate and make a relationship what it is. Don't forget those little things; savor them. Find joy in the little things and your relationship will prosper.

Whether we intend to or not, we are always communicating something. In the same way that we all have different hobbies and interests that engage us in life, we all have different styles of communicating with others. Some of us are very good at clearly expressing our thoughts, and others are not. With some, we listen more, and with others, we talk more. With some, we tend to be more open and have deeper conversations, and with others, we keep things more light-hearted. At different times, with the same people, we communicate differently. However, without effective communication, the world becomes very limited.

Communication is not just one thing; it's many things. It is easy to think of communication as just spoken words, but we also communicate with body language, facial expressions, in writing, eye contact, the tone and volume of our voices, attitude, and even in the way we dress. The physical environment conveys information as well. Signs communicate information as do decor, sound, and color. Think about the mood that an elegant restaurant creates. The dim lighting, formal clothing of the staff, and fancy decorations communicate that you should speak quietly and act politely instead of playing games, listening to music, or talking on the phone.

> **Communication**
>
> *Verbal Communication*
> Spoken words
>
> *Nonverbal Communication*
> Body language
> Gestures
> Environment
> Facial expressions
> Clothing

We communicate with others because it enables us to control, to some extent, what is going on in our lives. We can share feelings and ideas, give guidance and directions, ask for help, or express needs. When we have a hard time communicating with someone, we have trouble developing a relationship with him or her. We need relationships with our family, children, co-workers, community, pets, and people with dementia. We communicate in some way with everyone around us all day.

Communication disorders among people with dementia are often misunderstood and may go unrecognized for some time. Communication impairment can create difficulties between the person with dementia and his or her care partners, resulting (for the person with dementia) in becoming more dependent on others as well as increased stress for the care partners. These communication deficits can also lead to less participation in social activities and increased social withdrawal.

When communication is compromised, care partners often take over or provide excessive support during activities, such as bathing or dressing, unknowingly reinforcing dependence or unintentionally promoting aggressive behaviors. However, if you use effective communication strategies when interacting and helping someone with dementia, you will foster a better relationship with the person and facilitate independence for that individual.

A person with dementia still has the same needs as everyone else. The person wants to socialize, express needs, participate in hobbies, interact with family, be included in activities, teach and learn, and enjoy being asked for advice. The person has the same desire to contribute to the household or the community.

The need to communicate and be productive doesn't end once someone receives a diagnosis of dementia. A person who is just beginning to deal with cognitive impairment is often aware of difficulties in finding words and memories, and he or she often has an incredibly strong desire to connect with others to feel some sense of normalcy.

As the person struggles to communicate and remember daily information, he or she needs to have conversations and relationships that are successful. This is where you as a care partner can help. Your loved one needs positive reinforcement that they are valued. Although a person with dementia may not be able to contribute to conversations in exactly the ways they could before, there are still so many things the person *can* do. Care partners will have the most success when they concentrate thoughts on nurturing all that is still there instead of focusing on what is impaired.

Communicating with Someone with Dementia

Take a moment to imagine having a very uncomfortable sore on the end of your big toe. Every morning, you take a walk with your spouse. Every morning, the sore on your toe becomes aggravated, and then it throbs all day. Now, imagine that you can't think of the word *toe*, and you are having trouble expressing the feeling of pain to your spouse. How would you feel? What might you do? Most likely, you would feel frustrated, and maybe embarrassed or inadequate. Or worse yet, you might start refusing to go on the walk. You might use gestures and words that don't make sense to your spouse. In other words, your behaviors indicate that there is a problem or need you are trying to communicate.

Behaviors are a form of communication. The word *dementia* often carries a reputation for causing negative, bad, or disruptive behaviors. However, we would like to suggest that while they might be negative to us, they are often just the expression or communication by the person with dementia. Furthermore, when addressed properly, they are a mechanism for interactive communication between care partners and a loved one with dementia.

When we imagine ourselves in someone else's shoes and try to view the world through his or her eyes, we are better able to interpret the behaviors. Knowing the person well will help us, as care partners, figure out what the person is trying to tell us. If you are a professional care partner, make an effort to speak with the person's family and find out where the person lived, his or her hobbies and interests, their profession, and favorite foods. The more you can learn about this person, the more you will have to talk about, and the easier it will be to assist the person when they have difficulty communicating a need.

The First Step

> When interacting with people who have dementia, the rule of thumb should be: start by treating people with dementia the same as people without dementia and adapt your approach as necessary.

Begin by asking yourself why this behavior is happening. Is the person afraid? Hungry? Bored? In pain? Whenever we are asked to help problem-solve a situation in which a person with dementia is exhibiting "disruptive" behaviors, the first question we ask the care partner is "Why do you think this is happening?" The second question is addressed to the person with dementia. "What are you trying to do (leave house, empty all the milk containers, call the police, etc.)?" You would be surprised by how often these simple questions shed light and offer solutions to daily problems. Of course, sometimes the person doesn't know or cannot express why they are doing something. That's when we need to try to be the interpreter.

Often when responding to someone's behaviors, care partners react by removing the item that is being used inappropriately or by restricting movement because of safety concerns. This is not always the best solution for someone with dementia. For example, if your loved one tries to leave the house every morning and argues with you when you ask him or her to stay in the house, your immediate reaction might be to lock all the doors. Instead, ask, "Why is my wife leaving the house? Is there something in the house that is bothering her? Would she like to work in the garden? Would she like to go for a walk? In the past, was she in the habit of leaving for work or walking the dog right after breakfast?" Next, try testing some solutions. Rather than trying to restrict her from leaving the house, try scheduling a short walk every morning right after breakfast and time in the back yard after lunch.

Here is another example. Your husband is upsetting you because he fidgets with all of the kitchen appliances, clocks, alarm clocks, phones, mixers, etc., and he has already broken one alarm clock and a toaster. Your first instinct might be to put away all of the appliances and clocks out of sight. However, if you stop to consider why your husband might be doing this, you may come to the conclusion that he is bored. If he has always liked fixing things, maybe that is why he is doing so. It could be that he wants to feel useful or helpful. In any case, try setting up a card table in the kitchen or family room with items from the thrift store that your husband can "fix" for you. It would be wise to set up this space close to where the care partner spends time if safety is a concern.

Of course, some problems are not so simple to solve. Instead of removing objects or restricting movements, always look for a reason for the behavior and a way to let the person engage in a meaningful activity. Most behaviors are just a means of communicating a need that isn't met, and often the need is to be active, safe, useful, or busy.

Encouraging Socialization

Depending on the cause of a person's dementia, the ability to verbally communicate may take on different appearances. Some people may become very chatty, but others might not understand what they are saying. If the person has trouble finding the right words to communicate, he or she may become frustrated and speak less. The person may substitute one word for another word that isn't even related.

As a person with dementia begins to struggle with losing ideas for what to talk about or has difficulty processing conversations, he or she may become more isolated and withdrawn. In these cases, it is important to remember that the changes are occurring because of the disease process. The people without the disease are more capable of understanding and changing their approaches and responses.

Tips for Successful Communication

1. Be realistic in your expectations.
2. Be positive.
3. Listen carefully.
4. Ask one question at a time.
5. Ask yes-or-no questions.
6. Give choices, even if it seems insignificant.
7. Speak respectfully, using adult language.
8. Be aware of your body language, and pay attention to your partner's body language.
9. Use written cues and other visual aids.
10. Use touch.
11. Pay attention to "rambling" because it has meaning.
12. Verify comprehension during the conversation.
13. Avoid quizzing, arguing, or confronting.
14. Avoid saying *no* and other commands.
15. Use humor.
16. Speak *to* the person.

In spite of increasing communication deficits, people with dementia retain many functional communication abilities. Care partners can capitalize on the remaining communication strengths to help compensate for any lost communication abilities. As we have mentioned before, embrace what skills remain.

To better understand the communication behaviors of a person with dementia, care partners should think about what has changed *and* about what is preserved. Some of our suggestions may seem like common sense, and they are in a way. However, there are so many personal and professional demands on care partners that often we get caught up in completing the task at hand and forget about using some of these simple strategies to connect with the person in a meaningful way. The following suggestions should serve as a good reminder of the tools that you already have.

Always speak respectfully using adult language. If you are a professional care partner, using childlike speech or words such as *sweetie* will be viewed as negative by many older adults. A person with dementia is an adult with dementia, not a child. It is true that words such as *honey* or *darling* can convey affection, but there are other ways to express affection without belittling the person. You can smile and address the person by name and shake his or her hand. Family care partners should use whatever name or term of affection they have always called their loved one since it will be familiar to the person.

Keep the pitch of your voice low. Sometimes when a person doesn't immediately understand, there is a tendency to speak louder. Do you enjoy when someone shouts at you? Shouting distorts speech and will usually upset the person, making communication even more difficult. Speak in a warm, easygoing manner, and use the tone of voice that you would like people to use when speaking with you.

Be aware of body and facial gestures and expressions. People with dementia are aware of nonverbal messages, and they pay attention to them. Use these effectively as additional cues that may help someone process the information more accurately. You want the person to feel safe and comfortable, and you want them to trust you. In addition, pay attention to your partner's gestures and facial expressions because those nonverbal behaviors will communicate what they are not able to communicate with words. You may be able to tell if they are frustrated, didn't understand you, or are experiencing pain.

Watch someone's eyes to determine what is understood. A blank, empty look may indicate that they do not understand. Eye-to-eye contact means that they are paying attention. A smile with eye-to-eye contact may mean focused attention, interest in a topic being discussed, a little understanding, a feeling of comfort, or agreement and a willingness to do the activity. For example, in response to a request to get the newspaper for you, a smile with eye contact may be a sign of agreement, although you may need to point out the newspaper and start the person in the right direction.

Keep the conversation going. When you have a conversation with someone with dementia, it is your responsibility to keep that conversation going because he or she may have lost that ability. Introduce topics that the person enjoys and that are on his or her level of comprehension. Don't worry about whether the person's answers seem incorrect. Just enjoy the fact that the person is engaging with you. Providing choice questions is a very helpful strategy. A choice question is an inquiry phrased so the listener has a choice between two things. When you use a choice question, you are providing the information for the person to use in his or her answer.

"Bob, would you like soup or a sandwich?" is much easier for a person to answer than an open-ended question such as, "What would you like for lunch?" Once he makes a choice, you can add to the conversation by saying, "I'm having a sandwich too. I think I'll make egg salad today. That's my favorite." The person might then be encouraged to state his favorite or make another comment.

Ask yes-or-no questions. Questions that can be answered with a yes or no won't extend or prolong a conversation, but they are an effective means of giving someone a choice and keeping information simple. "Would you like soup?" You could also write the words "soup" and "sandwich" on index cards and show them to the person to determine what they prefer. Since reading is considered a preserved ability, it is another means of providing information that is likely to be successful. Written choices are also helpful because the person can point to the card if he or she is unable to respond verbally.

Don't ignore rambling. Keep in mind that rambling speech is communication too. Although it may seem like gibberish to you, listen for key words, gestures, and facial expressions to indicate what message the person is trying to convey. Pay close attention to the place or room where they are communicating. For example, if the person is in the kitchen or dining room, he or she may be hungry and asking for something to eat.

Avoid arguing, quizzing, or confronting. Engaging in these types of conversations will probably make the person angry or more confused. Often a person with dementia will ask to go home when they are already home, may look for someone who has passed away, or think they need to get on the bus and go to work. This can cause anxiety for you both and often escalates into a negative situation.

Acknowledge the person's reality. Accept the values, beliefs, and reality of the person suffering from dementia. The key is to agree with the person while using the conversation to encourage the person to do something else without realizing they are actually being redirected. For example, if an eighty-seven-year-old woman says that she needs to go home to take care of her five-year-old daughter, you could redirect her by saying, "I have a daughter too. She loves peanut butter and jelly sandwiches. Would you like to come into the kitchen to help me make a sandwich?" This distracts the person in a non-confrontational way and offers something meaningful to do.

Use a prompt to get the conversation going. A prompt is an easy way to gain someone's attention. Begin by making eye contact and saying the person's name or placing your hand on his or her shoulder. If you are giving an instruction, demonstrate exactly what you want the person to do before you ask him or her to do it. We like to tell the person, show the person, and then ask the person to show and tell us back. That way, they practice completing the activity, and we know the person has understood us. With some activities, such as brushing teeth or eating, actual hand-over-hand guidance will be needed to get the activity started.

Tips for Phrasing Your Requests in a Positive Approach

1. **Be impartial**. "Cups go on this shelf" is more effective than "I want you to be sure to keep the cups here."

2. **Be positive**. "Use your cane to keep you safe on our walk" is more effective than "Since you can't walk, you need to use this cane."
3. **Provide a reason**. "Please pick up your socks so the dog doesn't chew them" is more effective than "Put away your dirty socks."
4. **Provide a solution**. "Please move so Bert can see the television" is more effective than "Don't stand right in Bert's way."
5. **Provide awareness of consequences**. "When you wear sandals, your feet hurt" is more effective than "Don't wear sandals."
6. **Recognize emotions**. "I understand that you are not hungry, but food will give you energy. I enjoy when you eat breakfast with me" is more effective than "You must eat, or you'll be tired all day."

Using Memory Books to Facilitate Communication

One approach to helping a person with memory, cognition, and language problems is to use a memory book. Many studies have documented the effectiveness of memory books designed to provide the information that the person has trouble remembering.

First created by Michelle Bourgeois, a PhD and speech-language pathologist, memory books help stimulate conversation between people with dementia and their care partners. To help people who have trouble recalling names and places, memory books provide visual cues in the form of pictures and written text to help with these issues. Memory books have been found to help increase factual autobiographical statements and to decrease negative conversational comments, such as confused statements.

Memory books are a wonderful project to do with a loved one with dementia. You can easily make this an intergenerational project by including children and grandchildren. It is a nice way to connect the generations and learn about a loved one. It gives the person with dementia an opportunity to share information without having to remember all the facts. For more information, read *Memory and Communication Aids for People with Dementia* by Michelle S. Bourgeois.

How to Make a Memory Book

- Keep each page simple; use one phrase and one picture on each page.
- Use large-print and white paper with black lettering.
- Label pictures in the way in which the person would identify them.
- Put a photo of the person on the cover. Allow the person to choose the photo.
- Make sure it is meaningful and memorable so that when the person sees it, he or she will want to pick it up and look at the book.
- Include a daily schedule.

Remember that hand signals, gestures, pointing, drawing, showing pictures, and writing words helps to convey meaning. Be careful, however, that these do not cause distractions. Do one thing at a time. First try speech. If repeating the spoken message does not work, try to point. Smile at the person. Be sure to get the person's attention before pointing.

During the conversation, assess comprehension. The person with dementia should explain what he or she just heard or respond with a *yes* or *no* to direct questions about the communication.

As care partners, we need to work at finding as many ways as possible to help people maintain their communication skills for as long as possible. When they can no longer speak, we need to give them opportunities through gestures, facial expressions, and touch to make their needs known and to connect with others. Here is a story from our friend Katie about an experience with her mother, who has dementia. Katie blogs about what it is like to have multiple generations living together with someone who has dementia. You can read her stories at www.movinginwithdementia.com.

> *It was a typical family dinner at Mom and Dad's house. Six of the adult kids, four grandkids, and one hired care partner all sat around the table with Mom and Dad; Mom sat at the head of the table like always. Mom's Lewy body dementia has progressed so far in the past year that she is now physically similar to a paraplegic. She cannot move most parts of her body on her own, except moving her arms a bit up and down while they stay bent at a ninety-degree angle with her hands clenched, and she can move her head to look side to side. My sister sat next to my mom, carefully feeding her dinner, and I was at the other end of the long table. We were talking, laughing, and out of nowhere I hear Mom's voice, clear as ever: "I am over here dying, and you are all ignoring me."*
>
> *We all became silent for a moment. You see, Mom does not talk much anymore, and when she does speak, often her words are garbled. Yet sometimes she*

says a full sentence, bright and clear, and insightful. This was one of those times.

After a moment of silence, we said, "You are right, Mom. We are ignoring you," and so we started talking directly to her, involving her in the conversation. She sat for most of the rest of the meal not responding with more than the occasional smile, most often looking off to the side into space.

Communicating with our loved one with dementia is difficult at all stages. In the beginning, they ask lots of questions and repeat lots of stories. A bit later, they may argue with you about what you are telling them and not understand what you are saying. Then they may become paranoid and defiant, and you can't figure out how to communicate to them that opening a car door while driving is unsafe. In the late stages, they may start garbling their words and eventually stop talking altogether. At all of these points, I have heard people say that those with dementia do not know anything, they don't understand anything, or they just are not there anymore, so why try to communicate? I think we can see from my mom's statement at dinner that no matter what stage of dementia someone is in, they are still here, they still know who they are, and they still deserve dignity and respect.

In each stage of dementia, you need a different communication style. When Mom was having hallucinations, we did not argue with her or try to prove what she was seeing was not real. First, we would ask, "Why is this happening?" This simple question has helped me navigate how to communicate with Mom effectively at all stages of dementia. "Why is Mom seeing strangers in the house?" Finally, we realized that the large bay windows have a lot of glare, and they reflect your own image. This hallucination *was happening because Mom was seeing people's reflections in the window. So, we put up curtains.*

In the eight years we have been living with Mom's dementia, two and a half of which my husband, son, and I had the privilege to live with Mom and Dad, I have never felt like my mother was gone or inaccessible to me. I just needed to learn to communicate with her at whatever stage she is in.

In contrast to the dinner during which we did not model good communication, my nine-year-old son Jeffrey supported my mother with communication while working on an art project with Mom. He helped her create a notecard out of felt flower shapes. He showed her two different shapes and asked if she liked the blue one or the purple, and sometimes she could say, "blue." If she couldn't, he tried to notice if her eyes settled on one shape rather than another. Then he took the shapes she had chosen and placed one on the card and asked, "Do you like this here?" and she could reply "yes" or "no." He moved the pieces around until she liked them and glued them down for her. In this way, he gave a person who could barely talk or move, agency in her own life. My son's behavior told his grandmother that she had worth, dignity, and individuality at all stages in her life. We are always showing Mom that we know she is still here. She is the same woman whose favorite color has always been blue and who dedicated her life to her family, kids, and grandchildren.

During the card making, Mom said little and rarely looked at Jeffrey. In the end, Jeffrey showed her the finished card. She opened her eyes, smiled, and said, "It's pretty, honey." Clearly, Mom is with us when we take the time to be with her.

Remembering Takes Practice

Unfortunately, many people have the misguided belief that individuals with Alzheimer's disease or other dementias cannot learn new information. Often health care professionals feel that attempts to teach people with dementia to remember information is a waste of time. This assumption creates a self-fulfilling prophecy, ensuring that efforts to teach a person with dementia or change one's behaviors will fail. Fortunately, research over the past twenty years has shown that there are effective memory interventions for dementia. It's safe to assume that people with dementia *can* learn.

Benefits of Memory Practice

- Successfully recall information over longer periods of time.
- Can help someone remember behaviors and strategies.

Care partners should understand that individuals with memory deficits can actually remember some things well. Whether a person can use what they know or remember something learned depends a great deal on how care partners interact with the person. In our earlier discussion about memory in this chapter, we mentioned that the memory of *knowing that*, or procedural memory, is considered a preserved ability in Alzheimer's disease in particular. Trying these interventions with your loved one who has another type of dementia is advantageous with no negative side effects. Brush and many of her colleagues have conducted research and published articles and books about a learning technique called *Spaced Retrieval* that taps into procedural memory to help people retain and recall information.

Spaced Retrieval (SR) is an evidence-based intervention technique that provides a person with dementia-structured practice at remembering. SR is a procedure that involves selecting information or a behavior to be learned, telling the person the information, and then giving the person immediate practice at remembering. Practice at recalling the information is then prompted in expanding intervals of time. It can be used to help individuals lead more independent lives and can result in less repetitive questioning, better orientation, greater engagement in activities, improved appointment keeping, or safe ambulation. Achievement of these skills can promote independence and reduce anxiety.

Spaced Retrieval is practice at successfully recalling information over progressively longer intervals of time. The goal of the technique is retention of and an ability to recall information for a long time.

Think of information that your loved one would really like to remember but cannot. An example is remembering when someone is coming to visit. Your wife can tell time and remembers that her daughter comes to visit every day, but she always forgets the time of the visit and asks about it repeatedly. Let's walk through the procedure of helping her remember that her daughter visits at 4:00 p.m.

Practice at Remembering: The *Spaced Retrieval* Technique

1. Begin with a question for the target information and teach the person to recall the correct answer. "June, I

am going to help you remember when Emily comes to visit. Emily comes at 4:00. When does Emily visit?"

2. June responds, "4:00," and you reply, "Yes, that's right."
3. Let about thirty seconds pass. You can talk about or do anything you would like.
4. Then ask, "June, when does Emily visit?"
5. June responds, "4:00," and you reply, "Yes, that's right."
6. This time, let about one minute pass. You can talk about or do anything you would like.
7. Then ask, "June, when does Emily visit?"
8. June responds, "4:00," and you reply, "Yes, that's right."
9. Next, let about two minutes pass. You can talk about or do anything you would like.
10. Then ask, "June, when does Emily visit?"
11. June responds, "4:00," and you reply, "Yes, that's right."
12. Throughout the day, give June practice at remembering by gradually increasing the amount of time that passes in between practices (four minutes, eight minutes, sixteen minutes, etc.). Practice three to five intervals a few times a day each day until the person knows the answer automatically. You will find that she will stop asking the question repeatedly because she now knows the answer. If June were to make a mistake, give her the correct answer right away and then ask her immediately to recall it.
13. "June, when does Emily visit?"
14. June responds, "2:00" and you reply, "Actually, Emily visits at 4:00. When does Emily visit?"

This technique is called errorless learning. A person with dementia cannot recall personal episodes because of the impairment in *knowing that* or episodic memory; therefore, he or she cannot use the earlier information as a source for correcting himself or herself. The person must not be allowed to make errors in order to learn new information accurately. If errors are made, inaccurate learning will take place. Remember that if a recall failure occurs, the person is told the correct response and asked to repeat it. Then continue increasing the length of time between practices.

This technique can also be used to teach behaviors or procedures, such as going to the calendar or bulletin board to read the list of chores for the day, using a cane when walking, locking wheelchair brakes, putting glasses away in the same place every day. The procedure is the same except that in addition to practicing saying the information such as, "I put my glasses in their case," the person needs to practice the behavior at the same time. As a result, the practice involves saying the information *and* doing the behavior throughout the day.

The more we focus on enjoying what the person with dementia has to contribute, say, or do, the more enjoyment we will have in our day. It is so easy to become frustrated when someone is asking us the same question over and over, but using simple strategies can go a long way toward helping you connect and communicate with those in your care.

Understanding your loved one is doing the best he or she can and accepting that the communication will be different is the first step. Embrace the communication skills that are still strong to help compensate for those abilities that are lost, and know that your loved one still desperately wants and needs to communicate with you and with others in order to stay connected to the world.

Chapter 5

Creating Meaningful Time, Not Just Passing the Time

When you encourage someone, you build hope. When you build hope, you support dreams and celebrate achievements. People with dementia still have hopes and dreams and achievements. What can you celebrate today?

Paul was a very bright lawyer and adored his family. As he experienced the progression of his dementia, however, he became very lonely and longed for more companionship than his family could provide. However, as is the case with most families, his wife and daughter were convinced that Paul would resist having a companion. So Paul and his wife met Abby and me at a local coffee shop. Abby was an aspiring actress who excelled in all areas, but she needed more experience singing in front of others. Having just graduated from college, Abby was at the crossroads of "what's next in life." Paul loved opera and, while he confessed he could not sing, he loved to listen to music. Fortunately, he also couldn't help but give advice to others.

Our purpose in arranging this meeting was to manage the conversation in such a way that Paul would be comfortable spending time with Abby. After Paul and Abby seemed comfortable with each other, the plan was to suggest they get together because it seemed like they would enjoy each other's company. However, before I had the chance to say anything, Paul said to Abby, "Hey, why don't we do this? A few times a week, let's get together, and you can sing in front of me, and then we can talk about what you should do in life." His wife and I were in shock! We approached the situation thinking we had all the control, but in actuality, Paul, the man with dementia, took control. The outcome was better than we hoped for, and it was all his idea!

Establish Goals

Conventional wisdom says that people with dementia don't have goals. This is a myth. People with dementia do have goals. Have you ever noticed that a person with dementia always has a place to go or someone to meet? Despite whether these places or people exist anymore is irrelevant. Their desire emphasizes that he or she does have goals. One way to prove this point is to ask, "What would you like to accomplish today?" Take a minute, put this book down, and ask your loved one this question.

Welcome back! Now that you know that the person has goals, we can discuss how to set and accomplish these goals.

The first step is to distinguish between *realistic goals* and *unrealistic goals*. Here is where conflict may arise. Typically, when asked, the person with dementia will want to do something that's not realistic. He or she may say, "I want to go to work." The care partner often tries to bring the person from his or her "reality" to actual reality, which usually results in conflict. The person with dementia is left to do one of two things: move on by himself or herself or argue with the care partner. If the care partner responds in an argumentative manner, it only serves to escalate the situation.

As the care partner, you are the one who can change—not the person with dementia. Not because he or she doesn't want to, but because you are the one who has the power, the understanding, and the ability to recognize that there are two different "right" answers. In addition, when the frontal lobe of the brain is damaged (see chapter 2 to learn more about the parts of the brain), a person's ability to reason or make appropriate judgments can be impaired. When a person argues with a person with dementia, the person without the disease has an advantage and should not use it to challenge the person with dementia.

Lastly, it is important that the care partner recognize that some of the goals are unrealistic, but some of them will just look different once they are accomplished. In the latter case, the care partner needs to adjust his or her expectations and be prepared to roll with the punches. As you become comfortable, write down the goals of the person with dementia. It is good to refer to this list and see if he or she wants to change the goals at some point. You can write your goals as well and look at them together.

Goals of Person with Dementia	Goals of Care Partner
#1	#1
#2	#2
#3	#3

Give Up Control

As care partners, we become experts at trying to control every situation. We hope to minimize the unexpected, make life better for the person with dementia, and in the process, make our jobs easier. Actually though, trying to maintain control constantly can create a great deal of resistance and make everyone's life a little bit harder. Routine and structure are both very valuable, but they don't equate to control. Join us in an example.

> *Joyce was beginning to have some confusion and have trouble remembering conversations from ten minutes earlier, especially small talk. On occasion, she was burning meals and experiencing horrible, real-life dreams mid-day, which were ruining her afternoons. Her husband asked me to sit and talk with them. Joyce was surprisingly open about her situation and voiced her frustrations. Nick, being very self-disciplined, couldn't help but exert this same control toward Joyce.*
>
> *After our discussion about what was best for Joyce (yes, she was a part of the entire conversation), I asked her what her goals were to stay most engaged. She gave us three. The first was to embrace new friendships because at eighty-three years old, most of her friends had died or moved away. The second was to read books that were easier to follow rather than not read at all. The last was to play tennis one extra day a week (she was already playing two days a week). Her goals included socialization, cognitive strengthening, and physical exercise.*
>
> *Nick said, "Wow. I wouldn't have thought to ask her, but she came up with better goals than I would have."*

By asking the opinion of the person with dementia, you are giving him or her control, something we are all keenly aware of when someone takes it away. It is very common for a person with dementia to experience depression. However, how we treat the person is often a bigger contributor to the problem. While a person with dementia needs help, and may not be able to function as he or she did before being diagnosed, the care partner does not need us to take over his or her life. Unfortunately, this is often what we do without realizing it.

Points to Remember

- While it may not seem to you that they can answer questions correctly, don't look for a *right* answer.
- Ask questions that don't have a yes-or-no answer or the person will always say *no* because he or she might be feeling insecure or unsure. Instead, start by asking questions that give options. "Should we do the laundry or dust the furniture first?"
- Remember that the questions aren't just about the other person; they are about both of you. When it's time to eat, *both* of you should eat together, and when it is time for exercise, it is time for *both* of you to exercise. So often, care partners, aiming to maintain control, phrase suggestions in a directive manner. "You need some fresh air," or "You need to eat," or "You need to exercise," etc. It would be much more productive to say, "I would like some fresh air, would you come with me?" or "Should we walk around the neighborhood or go to the park?"

- A person with dementia enjoys spending time with loved ones and, in most cases, rises to the occasion to be able to do something together. They don't desire to watch TV all day, but it is often something they won't resist.

Small Changes, Big Successes

Bill was always a very athletic man. He played sports growing up and in college; afterward, he kept very active with tennis and golf. He would work out three times a week at his gym and then go to lunch with two of his gym buddies. As he became more forgetful and struggled to initiate his activities, he continued to go the gym and to lunch, but what happened at the gym changed.

In the beginning, Bill would exit the changing room and sit on a bench for just a short time. Then he would mount an exercise machine and complete his workout. As the months passed, his time on the bench became increasingly longer while his time exercising became shorter. One day, a staff member shyly approached him, unsure about what he was doing on the exercise bike, and Bill was sleeping.

When I called the gym to ask what services they had for a member who hypothetically had dementia, they asked, "Are you asking about Bill?" While I had intended to keep his name private, his condition clearly hadn't gone unnoticed by those who were involved in his daily life. To resolve the issue, his family bought Bill a personal trainer package so he had someone to get him started for the first thirty minutes of his workout. When they finished, his personal trainer would make sure

Bill used an exercise machine for the remaining half hour.

Bill is now working out again. This one change allowed him to resume his whole morning routine. While Bill complains that his personal trainer "is killing me," his face is filled with pride that his sons bought him the gift of a trainer. Bill is now up and out of the house three mornings a week, working out and socializing. Perhaps the silver lining is that Bill's wife has three mornings to herself.

So often, we struggle to think of what are we going to do on a particular day. Don't leave yourself exposed to last-minute decisions. A person with dementia will often wake up and, "What are we doing today?" Not being prepared only adds stress for the care partner at the very start of the day.

Have a plan for what you will do at least one day in advance. It is efficient and easy for everyone to be able to depend on a weekly schedule. This schedule is not set in stone, however, and it certainly can be changed if something comes up. The schedule should serve more as a guide. It should include the day of the week, the activity, the time of day, and who (if anyone) will be with the person with dementia.

When Making a Schedule

- Plan your day.
- Don't overcomplicate your day.
- Make sure one person is assigned to the person with dementia at all times.

- Bringing a person with dementia to family events is wonderful, but make sure that the person with dementia is a priority to one person in the group at all times.
- Make a schedule, and post it in the kitchen or family room. This allows visitors, care partners, family, and friends to know what to do at any given moment. It also allows the person with dementia some independence by knowing what to do for the day.

A Sample Schedule

Sunday	Monday	Tuesday	Wednesday	Thursday	Friday	Saturday
9:00 Breakfast 10:30 Church with Molly 11:45 Walk the dog with Molly 12:30 lunch with Molly 2:00 Family gathering at Lucy's 5:00 Dinner with Molly 6:30 TV News	9:00 Breakfast 10:00 read morning paper 11:00 Walk the dog with Molly 11:45 Prepare lunch with Molly 12:30 Lunch with Molly 2:00 Feed the ducks with Molly 3:30 Get ice cream with Molly 5:00 Dinner with Molly 6:30 TV News	9:00 Breakfast 10:00 Read morning paper 11:00 Walk the dog with Molly 11:45 Prepare lunch with Molly 12:30 Lunch with Molly 2:00 Art Therapy with Jan 3:30 Make smoothies with Molly 5:00 Dinner with Molly 6:30 TV News	9:00 Breakfast 10:00 Read morning paper 11:00 Walk the dog with Molly 11:45 Prepare lunch with Molly 12:30 Lunch with Molly 2:00 Walk the mall with Molly 3:30 Buy cookies with Molly 5:00 Dinner with Molly 6:30 TV News	9:00 Breakfast 10:00 Read morning paper 11:00 Walk the dog with Molly 11:45 Prepare lunch with Molly 12:30 Lunch with Molly 2:00 Yoga with Pat 3:30 Pick fresh vegetables with Molly 5:00 Dinner with Molly 6:30 TV News	9:00 Breakfast 10:00 Read morning paper 11:00 Walk the dog with Daniel 11:45 Prepare lunch with Daniel 12:30 Lunch with Daniel 2:00 Bridge game with the ladies 3:30 Tea and cookies with the ladies 5:00 Dinner with Daniel 6:30 TV News	9:00 Breakfast 10:00 Read morning paper 11:00 Walk the dog with Daniel 11:45 Prepare lunch with Daniel 12:30 Lunch with Daniel 2:00 Go to the park with grandkids 5:00 Dinner with Daniel 6:30 TV News

Use this blank calendar to plan your week. Change times to accommodate your schedule.

Sunday	Monday	Tuesday	Wednesday	Thursday	Friday	Saturday
9:00	9:00	9:00	9:00	9:00	9:00	9:00
10:00	10:00	10:00	10:00	10:00	10:00	10:00
11:00	11:00	11:00	11:00	11:00	11:00	11:00
11:45	11:45	11:45	11:45	11:45	11:45	11:45
12:30	12:30	12:30	12:30	12:30	12:30	12:30
2:00	2:00	2:00	2:00	2:00	2:00	2:00
3:30	3:30	3:30	3:30	3:30	3:30	3:30
5:00	5:00	5:00	5:00	5:00	5:00	5:00
6:30	6:30	6:30	6:30	6:30	6:30	6:30

Socialization is a key factor to promoting well-being. However, the stress of being with new people can cause insecurity. It is critical that the person with dementia be reassured regularly that they are going to be successful in making new friends. When the person with dementia is going to do something without his or her primary care partner or the person with which they are most secure, it is good to remind him or her that the meeting or event will only be for a short time. Assure the person that you are looking forward to seeing him or her again. Before he or she leaves the house, give the person a note that says you will be back in a short time.

Since you may feel like you are in this alone, invite your friends and family to be part of your care team. Depending on their understanding and comfort level with the disease, they may not be proactive in asking you how they can support you. Here are some guidelines for how to include friends and family.

- Start by telling them that Michael has dementia, cognitive impairment, Alzheimer's disease, etc. Below is a sample letter to friends and family.
- Ask them what they like to do with Michael, and then ask if they are still comfortable doing so. If not, ask if they would mind if you gave them some suggestions. They can do what they have always done, or you can give them a specific project, such as going food shopping (give them a list) or taking the dog for a walk.
- When they finish, ask if they would be willing to help you again. If so, put a date on the calendar.

More simple than you expected, right?

Dear Friends,

As you may or may not know, Michael has been diagnosed with Alzheimer's disease.

Some of you have asked what you can do to help, so I thought it best to respond to everyone.

Alzheimer's disease is a type of dementia that causes cognitive impairment. Cognitive impairment involves problems with complex tasks, language, thinking, and judgment that are greater than normal age-related changes. Among other things, the disease causes short-term memory loss and intermittent confusion.

According to our dementia coach, the more we can keep Michael engaged, the more we may be able to slow the progression of his symptoms and improve his quality of life. This is where you come in. Please continue to call Michael and to visit him. He still talks about you. You are still an important part of his life, and he will be so glad to hear from you and continue your friendship.

If Michael gets confused during your conversation, he may say something that might not fit in with how you remember it. Please don't argue, but don't stop talking either. You may not understand what he is trying to say, but assure him that you understand and remind him again of good memories.

When you are in the area, we would love to have you stay with us. If that is not possible, perhaps we can have dinner or do something else together. Michael may forget to tell me of any plans you make with him, so it would be helpful if you kept me in the loop.

We are all doing spring cleaning. As you find old pictures, please send us a copy and remind us of the details behind it (as much as you can). We would love to relive the moment with you.

I know that you care deeply for Michael, and I so much appreciate any interaction you continue to have with him. Thank you for being such a dear friend.

Make It Happen!

A patient came through the emergency room at a local hospital, and during her stay proved to be agitated, aggressive, and at times combative. Adele was moved to one of the acute care floors and was met by Donna, a certified nursing assistant who had recently finished a course in best-care practices for people with dementia. Adele was wheeled down the hall, her arms tied to the bed, when Donna met her. Donna thought, Excellent, let's try out my new skills.

The first thing she did was untie Adele. After that, when Adele wanted to get up and look out the window, Donna walked with her. When Adele was ready to eat, Donna served her. When Adele wanted to talk, Donna listened. When Adele wanted things quiet, Donna was quiet. Adele never exhibited any of the behavior described when she was in the ER. Furthermore, during Adele's six-week stay in the hospital, she never exhibited any of these behaviors. All the other staff members talked about what a difference Donna's care made. Donna shared what she had learned with the staff.

It's important to know how to deal effectively with a person who has dementia, but there comes a time when you have to start doing it. You need to sit and listen to what the person with dementia has to say. When the person asks why you are looking at him or her, you can say, "I want to hear what you have to say." When you want the person to go for a walk, ask him or her to join you. Don't ever say anything about why walking is healthy; the person is going for *you*. Try it!

Take a Step Back

> *Focus on abilities rather than impairments*

Trial and error (and success) should be your guide. When you find that something didn't work, consider it a success because you now know something not to do. Expect and accept that things will change. It is also all right if the person with dementia decides to keep things just the way they are.

Keep a list of what works and what doesn't. Refer to it often, and don't hesitate to share it with the person who has dementia. The person will, at times, tell you that something that he or she said no to should be on the yes list. Don't argue. Just remind the person that he or she said no previously, and commend them for wanting to try something new. We are all free to change our minds—and so is a person with dementia.

Meaningful Activities

Now that we have talked about including the person with dementia in establishing daily routines and have discussed creating a schedule ahead of time, the last step is what to put on the schedule. In addition to the normal routine that works for the person with dementia, below is a list of interesting activities.

Art. Art is proven intervention to help those with dementia to relax and gain confidence, and it should be encouraged whenever possible. Whether you sign the person up for a drawing class at a local community college or have a high school or college art student visit your home, this activity can be very rewarding.

- To find an artist, call your local high school or college and ask to speak with the art teacher. Ask them if they have any students who might be interested in doing art with someone with memory impairment. Make sure you, the care partner, are present when the artist first meets your loved one so that everyone will be comfortable. The young person might be uneasy at first.

20 Activities to Do in a Pinch

- Play solitaire
- Jigsaw puzzles
- Sort and/or fold laundry
- Cut coupons
- Wash and cut up fruit and vegetables
- Water indoor and outdoor plants
- Play music
- Listen to an audiobook
- Sort silverware
- Reading material
- Craft or hobby projects
- Word searches
- Photo albums
- Arrange fresh flowers
- Crochet or knit
- Fill the bird feeder
- Exercise video
- Make the bed
- Read jokes out loud
- Search for topics of interest on the Internet

- Call a local art school to see how they can work together with you.

- Contact local art therapy programs at the university level, and inquire about students who would be willing to engage your loved one.

- Contact the Global Alliance for Arts and Health (www.thesah.org), and ask for the contact information of an artist in your area who works with older adults.

Reading. Yes, a person with dementia can often read for a long time. Reading is considered a preserved ability in dementia. The goal is not to see him or her read to understand as he or she once did or to see if he or she remembers and comprehends the text. The goal is to enjoy the act of reading. If reading continues, he or she will be able to maintain this ability for a longer period of time. We recommend that grandchildren ask a grandparent with dementia to read to them when they visit. These books are easier to read and the grandchildren will be more receptive.

- Use the Quick Reading Check in the appendix to see which type size is best for the person with dementia. Once this is determined, print out articles, advice columns, or short stories in the same type size. Make sure to ask the person with dementia if they are enjoying what they are reading since interests change from time to time.

- Writing and reading. Have grandchildren become pen pals with their grandparents who have dementia. If done by e-mail, print out the e-mails so the person with dementia can read the letters more frequently, especially as short-term memory becomes shorter.

Church, Temple, Religion. People with dementia respond very well to religion that they have always practiced or even slightly practiced during their lives. Whether it is something as simple as reading the Bible at home, singing hymns, or visiting a church or temple regularly, a person with dementia will often thrive in this setting. Some people are happy just to be in spiritual settings, and they might not be in any of the places listed above. If this is the case, make this part of your regular routine. Suggestions to make the spiritual life of a person with dementia more accessible are:

- Tell the people you are closest with at church or temple about your loved one's diagnosis. They can be available to help and give you some needed relief at the same time.

- Give your loved one something to do at the service such as passing out programs or greeting people when they arrive.

Write out his or her life story. Using pictures and a photo album, go through your pictures, one at a time, and discuss the picture. Write a simple story, using just a few sentences or phrases, and include it with the picture on one page in the album. If the pictures are labeled with names, there can be more than one picture on a page. The book will be a great resource throughout the course of the disease. It will be a joy for the person with dementia to look through and for all care partners who come through his or her life.

Cats and Dogs. Call your local animal shelter or humane society to inquire about volunteering. Most organizations need volunteers to help brush the animals or put out fresh water. These are simple tasks, but it can be very rewarding to be part of this care. Be careful not to take too many animals home. One care home bakes fresh dog biscuits and delivers them every other week to the dogs. The visits are loved by all!

Volunteer. Instead of looking for fun and entertaining things to do, find settings where the person with dementia is needed. Some suggestions include the local park system, soup kitchens, food pantries, or libraries. Contact your local church or temple and ask what volunteer work is available. It might be something as simple as collating the Sunday bulletin.

Music. A great deal of research has been done that validates the positive effects that music has for people with dementia. Contact local music therapy programs at colleges for students to engage with your loved one. Many students will be willing to do this for free to gain experience.

- Make music a part of your everyday life. Identify which music helps keep your loved one calm, and play it when he or she tends to get anxious or agitated.

- Music can also be a successful intervention during care. Play the person's favorite music during bathing, dressing, or getting ready for bed.

Exercise. This is one of the best things that *all* of us can do to reduce stress, stay healthy, and clear our heads. Research has shown that the same outcomes are true for people with dementia. The recommended exercise routine is to get at least thirty minutes of exercise, five days a week. This is a good habit for a person with dementia as well as his or her care partners.

This exercise can take place in a gym—or it can be as simple as a walk around the block. There are also exercise videos available for people who need to stay seated while exercising. These can be found online. If you or your loved one have other health concerns, consult your physician about what exercise will be most beneficial for you.

- It is beneficial to exercise in the afternoon in order to help relieve anxiety and agitation that is often common in the late afternoon or early evening. Regular exercise usually has a positive effect on sleep patterns as well.

- Often, a person with dementia doesn't want to or will say no when asked to exercise. It is important that this time is a bonding time rather than something they have to do. In one example, the husband with dementia attends a gym where he works out a number of days a week. However, his wife wanted to walk in the evenings because it made her feel better. When she told him he had to go, he refused. When she asked him to join her because she wanted his company, he would go willingly (most of the time).

- Adopt a local pet in the neighborhood and become the dog walker.

- Invite a local child in the neighborhood to go for a walk (when there is a care partner present).

- Ask a high school student or young person to walk daily with this person.

- Young men can be a great motivator for an older man. Post an ad in the local fitness center to recruit a young man to join the person with dementia to exercise.

- As a person with dementia becomes weak, the common course of action is to try to keep him or her seated as much as possible to reduce the risk of falling. However, this actually increases weakness and makes one's balance even more unstable. If your loved one is weak or unstable, talk to a physician and get a referral for a physical therapist. The physical therapist will do an evaluation, provide an appropriate set of exercises, and prescribe a walker or other assistive device, if needed. There are outpatient and home health physical therapists available in most areas. This is a great service since it physically helps the person with dementia, gives the person with dementia a visitor, and provides a respite for the care partner.

- It's common that as people progress through the disease, they become less motivated to get up and move around. Creating an exercise routine early in the disease process will help the person with dementia to remain stronger, which will also decrease the risk of falling. Some people will walk incessantly during the middle to later stages of the disease. There is no evidence, however, that maintaining an exercise program early on results in the incessant walking.

Give the person a project to do (for example, painting the birdhouse) or have the person accompany a friend or family member to the store. It needs to be very specific so that it actually helps the primary care partner and gives purpose to the person with dementia and his or her companion.

Local Adult Day Centers. Research local *social model day programs*. These programs will provide socialization and a day filled with activities so that the person with dementia can enjoy the day. Usually, *social model day programs* do not provide personal care or toileting. However, if the person with dementia needs these services, then look for a *medical model day program*.

Look at senior day centers and memory cafés. These programs help the people with dementia stay socially engaged, meet new people, and keep engaged in dealing with new things.

People with dementia should participate in meaningful activities as often as possible. When people are happy and doing things they love, they are not displaying negative or inappropriate behaviors. Keep in mind that the things on the schedule are not just for the person with dementia; they are also for the care partner. Both should enjoy mid-day snacks, going for walks, or spending time with grandkids. Don't discount the time because it is not how you would have liked it to be. You will miss out on what your loved one with dementia has to offer—as well as what you are doing.

When Visiting Your Loved One

- Expect good things—despite what has always been, don't expect your loved one to be in a bad mood or assume that he or she will get upset with you. Expect the person to be happy to see you, and likewise, be happy to see him or her.
- Bring things to focus on, do, or look at.
- Start with short visits, between fifteen and thirty minutes (and less is okay too). The person won't remember the amount of time. The goal is to have a good experience, not a long time together.
- Visit during meal times or activities you know your loved one enjoys. Make friends with other residents, and tell them nice things about your loved one.
- Don't visit in the person's room because you will become isolated.
- When the person starts asking to go home, answer kindly and then leave. Usually these conversations will wear you out, and the person probably won't remember what you say. There is nothing to be gained by saying it over and over.
- Assure the person at all times that you will only do what is in his or her best interest.
- When you leave, don't make a big deal about it. Be sure to include that you will see them again. "I will see you later, Mom. I have to run to the store to get my errands done before it gets too late. I had a nice time with you, and I'm looking forward to seeing you soon!"

Chapter 6

Making the Home Safe and Supportive

Home is not a house or a certain town. It is wherever the people who love you are, whenever you are together. The moments spent together build upon one another like a stone foundation for a house. You can take that with you for your entire life, wherever you may go.

If you were to ask a hundred people how and where they would like to live during their older years, nearly everyone would say, "I want to be as independent as possible, and I want to live in my home." People rarely reply, "I hope I live in a nursing home."

One morning, I was working with a gentleman with early-stage Alzheimer's disease. I asked him to share the three most important things that I needed to know about his care as he advanced through the disease. He didn't tell me about his medication or even talk about his illness. He said, "I want to eat pizza, go fishing, and be able to play with my grandchildren."

It was my job to help his family figure out how to support these wishes so he could continue to do the things that were important to him.

Another client with dementia said, "I want to stay right here, tend to my plants, and take long walks in the woods."

These are simple requests of people wanting to carry on with life as usual, but for someone with Alzheimer's disease or a related dementia, life becomes confusing. Even one's own home can add to that confusion if the right care isn't taken to create a supportive home environment. How can we make daily life less challenging at home?

Here is an example that our friend Katie shared with us from her experience taking care of her mother at home.

> *There are many ways the environment can affect a person with dementia. When my husband, son, and I lived with my parents, we watched Mom progress from early to mid-stage dementia, then close to late stage. We did not know as much about dementia then as we do now. I remember it was hard for us, particularly for a seven-year-old boy, to understand why leaving a game out on the kitchen table was such a problem for Mom. Now we know that too much clutter is confusing for people with dementia, and simple things, like keeping common areas looking consistent every day, is very soothing to our loved ones.*
>
> *Items such as a new throw rug are foreign and confusing (not to mention a potential fall hazard), and wood cabinets with wood handles are too difficult to see. There are many environmental changes you can make to help your loved one simply by adding contrast, such as changing the wooden cabinet handles to red handles.*
>
> *Creating templates for items in the house can also be a big help. For instance, Mom always liked to set the table, but eventually she could not remember where the plates, cups, napkins, and silverware went. With Mom, we traced place settings onto large placemat-sized pieces of paper that we laminated. We put the placemats out, and then Mom was able to set the table by matching up the items to the outline on the placemat. With this simple template, we were able to give Mom back something that she thought she had lost. She was still able to contribute to her favorite family time, dinner, by setting the table.*

Organization Establishes Calmness

Have you ever lost your car keys? It's a silly question; of course, you have. We have all lost our car keys, cell phones, purses, or wallets at least once, if not many times, at some point in our lives. Everything needs a home. Having a home for these frequently used items helps all of us, not just people with dementia. People with dementia experience a reduction in the ability to process stimulation. As a result, a home environment with significant amounts of clutter can be over-stimulating and create difficulties in locating needed items, such as phones or wallets, which can lead to frustration and anxiety.

Visual organization means that commonly used items are clearly visible and that containers have prominently displayed labels. Clean up any clutter, and visually organize the environment by giving everything a home. Organizing items by category, such as putting the cup, toothpaste, and toothbrush together in one place, can serve as a useful reminder. Placing a labeled basket or other container by the door for keys or mail reduces the likelihood that these items will be misplaced. Labeling the kitchen cabinets with a list of contents will help the person with dementia find things more easily in the kitchen.

Memory Centers Produce Self-Dependence

Rather than putting excess demands on the impaired memory of someone with dementia, help the person by compensating for his or her losses. Create a memory center in your home. With practice, it will become the go-to place for important information such as the time, date, lists of things to do, daily schedules, and visitors for the day. One thing to keep in mind is that many people have a tendency to make this area very cluttered with post-it notes, lists, and photos. The memory center needs to strike a balance between providing the needed information and not looking visually cluttered.

Items to Place in Your Memory Center

- Large, easy-to-read digital clock or a large analog clock with a white face and black numbers. Look for an analog clock with Arabic numbers because they are easier to read than Roman numerals. If you aren't sure which to choose (digital or analog), pick the type of clock that your loved one is accustomed to using. You can also show the person each clock, one at a time, and ask him or her to tell you the time. If the response time for one of them is quicker, easier, or more automatic, choose that type of clock to hang in the memory center.

- Simple, large wall calendar with minimal designs or pictures. Many catalogs and office supply stores have memo boards with dry erase surfaces that already have a place for a calendar, notes, and daily schedules.

- Telephone. Many phones are designed for older adults and/or for people with hearing loss. It may be helpful to purchase a phone that is equipped with speakerphone because it allows a person with a hearing aid to use the phone without the risk of feedback. Phones with large buttons are ideal for people with low vision or limited fine motor abilities. There are also phones with memory buttons that can be preprogrammed and dialed with the touch of just one button. This is ideal for people with mild memory problems. Picture phones have room for a picture of the person next to the memory dial button. This is best for people with significant memory issues or limited literacy.

- Notebook and pens.
- Emergency information. Ambulance, fire, and police station numbers should be posted in large print.

Routines Provide Predictability

Pick a routine—and then stick to it. People with dementia will have less anxiety and confusion throughout the day if the daily routine is consistent. Find a flow for the day that is comfortable for your lifestyle, and stick to it. Don't plan too much. Keep in mind that someone with dementia will not be able to keep up the pace of a hectic day as he or she may have been able to earlier in life. For example, don't try to squeeze two or three appointments into one day. Instead, make one appointment for each day.

When daily routines are consistent, a person with dementia will learn the pattern of the day and will know what to expect, which will trigger the correct patterns of behavior. Certainly, there are unexpected events that pop into our lives that are

At Home

relaxed and comfortable
at ease
in harmony with the surroundings
on familiar ground

from *Merriam-Webster Dictionary*

beyond our control, and we need to be flexible and adjust our schedules. However, you will find that by providing structure and routine for someone with dementia, you are providing a sense of order that can be calming for the person. When you leave your loved one with someone else for the morning, afternoon, or an entire day, fully inform the care partner about the schedule so they can stick to the routine too.

Post a dry erase board by your memory center with the daily schedule, and give the person with dementia practice reviewing the board to find out what is next for the day (see the "Staying Engaged" chapter for Practice at Remembering).

One family member truly embraced this suggestion and developed a daily schedule for his wife. The schedule Jim created for Renee included time for hobbies, relaxing, and chores. When we met with Jim to follow up and see how the suggestion was working, he was very pleased, with one exception. Renee never unloaded the dishwasher when it was her turn. She would complete everything else on the schedule except for that.

We asked Jim why he thought Renee wasn't unloading the dishwasher.

He replied, "Well, she has dementia. She probably just forgets to do it."

We said, "Renee, Jim noticed that when the schedule says it's your turn to unload the dishwasher, you haven't been doing it. Why is that?"

Renee promptly responded, "I have always hated unloading the dishwasher. If I cook, he should clean up!" Renee reminded us of something important: people with dementia are still people with likes and dislikes. It is always harder for someone with dementia to do something they have never liked or have never done before than to do something they have always enjoyed.

Home Modifications Compensate for Deficits

Modifying the home environment can improve safety, promote independence, and ease the care giving. Home modifications are important for helping people with dementia. Examples of home modifications for someone in a wheelchair include adding a ramp into the house, low-hanging bars in closets, or grab bars in bathrooms. Examples of home modifications for someone with dementia may include labels on items, increased lighting, or increased contrast at the dining table.

The best modifications are created to take full advantage of a person's ability to continue to participate in daily activities and chores for as long as possible because everyone likes to feel productive and useful. Since most types of dementia are progressive (the symptoms get worse over time), a home modification that works today may not work the next month. Try not to become frustrated if that happens. Instead, recognize part of living with dementia means that you may need to make adjustments to your home space and routine as time goes on.

We are all unique; don't assume that everyone with dementia is the same. A home modification or intervention that works for one person may not work for another. Solutions to problems related to dementia always have to be customized to the situation or individual, the care partner, and the home. Make one modification to the home at a time. Making substantial changes that require the person to do a task in a totally different manner is likely to be overwhelming and can cause a significant agitation or confusion.

Some modifications are simple and do not require any special expertise, but other modifications require a skilled contractor. The National Association of Home Builders offers a certification called Certified Aging-in-Place Specialist. A

Certified Aging-in-Place Specialist has been trained in the unique needs of the older adult population, aging-in-place home modifications, common remodeling projects, and solutions to common barriers. The organization's website has a resource that enables consumers to find remodelers or contractors who specialize in the aging-in-place market.

Home modifications for people with dementia are usually made to compensate for memory, vision, and hearing impairments in the early to mid-stages, and to compensate for mobility and more significant cognitive impairments in the later stages of the disease.

These visual challenges include problems with contrast and depth perception and difficulty judging colors. Contrast helps us distinguish one item from another. Loss of contrast perception is a decreased ability to see the edges of things when they are the same color as what is around them. One place where loss of contrast perception is a common problem is in the bathroom, which often has a white or light floor, white toilet, and maybe even white or light-colored walls.

Depth perception is the visual ability to judge how far away things are as well as to be able to see things as three-dimensional objects. Loss of depth perception creates an effect that can cause difficulty going up and down stairs, reaching for objects, or sitting. While color perception declines with age for everyone, people with Alzheimer's disease or a related form of dementia exhibit a greater loss. Blues, blue-greens, and blue-violets often look the same. Red stands out the most, making red items easier for people with dementia to see.

When these visual abilities are disrupted, it is very stressful for people to make sense of any environment. When people do not see well, they become easily disoriented. Imagine how upsetting and frightening it is for people when their vision makes them see pieces or parts of things. For visual challenges, home modifications can help compensate for common visual deficits.

The warning signs for declining vision include repeatedly walking into objects, bruises on limbs, and unusual behaviors, such as putting lotion on a toothbrush. Families should not automatically assume these behaviors are caused by cognitive deficits, but they should check to see whether they are related to vision loss. Since a person with dementia has impaired communication skills, he or she may not inform anyone about changes in vision.

Suggestions for Home Modifications

Since each person with dementia is unique and every home is different, not all the modifications suggested will apply in your situation. In fact, many may not be necessary at all. The tips below take all causes of dementia into consideration. Use this list as a guide, and adapt the suggestions as needed.

Some of the suggestions related to safety involve storing knives, tools, appliances, cleaners, etc., in locked cabinets. This does not mean that your loved one should have access to nothing or that everything should be locked up. In fact, we believe that everyone should live in the least restrictive environment possible. For example, if your loved one does not put objects such as forks or pencils in the electrical outlets, you do not need to install outlet covers. If your loved one enjoys cooking for a hobby and can safely cut and peel vegetables, then by all means, encourage it. However, if your loved one begins putting eye drops in his or her mouth, you should place the eye drops in a locked cabinet.

Safety in and around the Home

- Use bells on the door, motion sensors that turn on lights or alerts, or other notification systems that alert the care partner when someone has gone outside.

- Increase lighting coming in and out of the house by adding lamps or motion-activated lighting to ensure that people can see where they are going.

- Add reflective tape strips on stair edges to make stairs more visible.

- Remove obstacles, such as mats and flowerpots, to minimize risk of falls on or by the stairs.

- Install grab bars and a raised toilet seat to help the individual with dementia and care partners so they don't have to lift the person on and off the toilet.

- Add grab bars inside and outside the tub and a non-skid surface in the tub to reduce the chance of falls. Add colored tape on the edge of the tub or shower curb to increase contrast and make the tub edge more visible.

- Lower the water temperature, install an anti-scald valve, and remove the drain plug from the sink and/or tub to prevent burns and/or floods.

- Camouflage features that attract someone to the door by covering doorknobs and locks or painting the door to match the walls. To discourage someone who often wants to leave the house, make sure that he or she gets plenty of outside exercise whenever possible. Also try posting "do not enter signs" on doorways, removing doorknobs, using gates or furniture to block access, or installing complicated locks.

- Remove or disable automatic locks on storm and screen doors so that the person does not get locked out of the house. Store an extra set of house keys somewhere safe but accessible outside the house.

- Clearly mark pathways, and use fencing to mark the perimeter of your property to avoid wandering. Installing locks on gates or keeping people with dementia on a deck or porch may also be necessary.

- Provide an identification or GPS bracelet in case of wandering.

- Label clothes with your loved one's name in case he or she gets lost.

- Place an identification card in your loved one's wallet along with a note describing his or her condition.

- Notify the local police and neighbors of the person's dementia and tendency to wander.

- Put decals on glass doors to make them more visible and prevent someone from walking into the glass.

- Swimming pools should be fenced in to prevent injury or drowning.

- Install magnetic locking systems or childproof locks on a few drawers or cabinets in the kitchen that are out of the way or rarely used.
- Store sharp knives, food processor blades, and kitchen appliances that might start a fire, such as a toaster oven, in these locked cabinets.
- Store tools in locked toolboxes.
- Remove firearms from home or store in a gun safe.
- Use an electric razor to prevent accidents while shaving.
- Store daily medications in a labeled pill box and the rest in a locked cabinet.
- Store all cleansers, chemicals, insecticides, fertilizers, paint, etc., in a locked cabinet to prevent accidental ingestion.
- Use colored switch plate covers that contrast with the walls to make it easier to find the light switches.
- Install childproof outlet covers.
- Install smoke detectors, and make sure that fire extinguishers are easily accessible.
- Remove dials on stoves, and place them in a locked drawer.

Improving Freedom of Movement

- Build a ramp to the front and back doors of your house to accommodate wheelchairs for people with reduced mobility.
- Install handrails in hallways and stairways to provide stability.
- Install a gate on the stairway to prevent falls.
- Install locks on the door to the basement to prevent falls or avoid potentially dangerous areas.
- Increase light levels in stairs and hallways by adding additional ceiling fixtures or wall sconces.
- Add non-skid strips to the stairs, or tape or paint stair edges to increase visibility.
- Use a shower chair or tub seat for bathing.
- Remove throw rugs that might trip an unstable walker.
- Remove or move low furniture, such as stools or coffee tables, which might not be seen and could pose a tripping hazard.
- Keep a clear path in the center of rooms so everyone can walk without bumping into or stepping over things.
- Use only non-skid mats in bathrooms, bathtubs, and showers.

- Use nightlights in hallways, bedrooms, and bathrooms.

Assisting with Personal Care and Daily Activities

- Post simple, large-print reminders about washing (e.g., labeling hot and cold on faucet, putting soap and shampoo in plain sight) to encourage independent personal care.

- Create reminders about toileting, such as a sign on the bathroom door. Or keep the door open to provide visual cueing and promote continence.

- Change the color of the toilet seat to maximize contrast against the toilet bowl. Paint the wall behind the toilet so it contrasts with the toilet and toilet paper, making it easier to find.

- Provide index cards or a small poster with the steps for toileting written out.

- Outline the sink in colored tape to distinguish it from the wall.

- Label the closet and/or dresser with the person's name and the items to be found in each drawer.

- Use wire baskets for storing clothing to make it easier to see.

- Install lighting in the closets to make it easier to locate clothing.

- If more than one person provides care, post a list of specific responsibilities that each care partner should perform, and communicate regularly with other care partners to help ensure the best care.
- Place clocks in frequently used rooms to help the person orient easily to the time of day.
- Eliminate shiny, glaring surfaces that might worsen depth-perception problems and cause confusion.
- Use reflector tape on floors or walls to help your loved one find his or her way.
- Keep personal care items in the same place all the time to provide as much consistency as possible.
- Simplify the task of getting dressed by arranging clothes on the bed in the order in which they should be donned. Give the person a choice of two outfits, and let him or her choose which one to wear.
- Use grooming tools such a hairbrushes and toothbrushes with curved handles that have been specifically designed for people with motor impairments to facilitate independence.
- Use an automatic dial telephone so the person can make calls independently.
- Keep a portable toilet available to enable a person with incontinence to reach a toilet easily from any part of the home.

- Prepare food in portions that can be easily eaten with fingers, and provide straws when serving liquids to help your loved one eat successfully without assistance.

- Use a vinyl tablecloth that can be easily cleaned to help make messy eating less troublesome.

Chapter 7

Taking Care of Yourself

While this disease can have devastating effects on your loved one, it is important to adjust your expectations and find joy in smaller, daily successes. This will help you, the care partner, not be as overwhelmed, frustrated, and disappointed.

Dementia not only affects those diagnosed with it; it also impacts all those involved in that person's life. Most resources focus on the care of the person with the disease, but care partners are also significantly affected by the disease and need to be cognizant of its effects on them so they can take the necessary steps to stay healthy—both physically and emotionally—in order to better care for their loved ones.

It is important, as a care partner, to adjust your expectations in order to find joy in smaller, daily successes. This will help you avoid feeling overwhelmed, frustrated, and disappointed. Despite this, frustration, disappointment, anger, and many other emotions might eventually surface—and quite understandably. This chapter will address some of these emotions and how care partners can work toward helping themselves work through them.

Overcoming Guilt

> *Roy, a former family physician, was a quiet, highly intelligent man. He was a wiz at history and an avid reader. He was diagnosed with Alzheimer's disease. After a few years, his wife began bringing him to an adult day program once a week, which took place inside of a memory care assisted living center.*
>
> *His mornings would start with a workout in the gym with a staff member. Then he would join the group for the day. Despite Sugar's anticipation that he would resist going, he actually enjoyed it. She enrolled him in the program three times a week. After four months of attending, as they were leaving, he said, "Would it be okay with you if I slept here all week and just came home on the weekends?" Sugar breathed a sigh of relief.*

Many people who care for a loved one with dementia experience a roller coaster of emotions. It is sad to watch someone you love change, and it is also sad to see the reactive change in us. We often feel that we can't do enough, and this guilt is only outweighed by the guilt of not wanting to be in the caregiving role in the first place, which pulls at us and creates a terrible game of emotional tug-of-war.

That is when care partners for people with dementia often begin to struggle emotionally. The changes in the person with dementia are gradual, and most don't affect the physical appearance of the person diagnosed, especially early on. Care partners feel guilty about needing a break because they feel like they are letting their loved ones down. For instance, if your husband asks to go to the store with you and then stays in the kitchen while you cook and continuously asks what you are doing, you might become very annoyed.

Early on in the disease process, care partners are not aware that the disease causes this behavior, and they argue with the person or express frustration.

The problem is that we can't see the damaged brain, but it is there. If your husband had a huge hole in the side of his head, it would be a reminder of why he is feeling insecure or repeats the same question. If your wife had a stroke and became paralyzed, your family would probably be open to accepting care. For people with short-term memory loss, families feel that they should be able to manage the situation on their own.

Care partners often burden themselves with a long list of self-imposed faults that are either imagined or unavoidable. Rather than treating themselves with compassion, care partners tend to beat themselves up and say, "I shouldn't lose my temper with someone who has dementia," "If I could take better care of my husband, he wouldn't have to live in a nursing home," or "I should stay home with my wife instead of playing a round of golf with my friends." These feelings of guilt stem from doing or saying what you believe is the wrong thing, not doing what you think is enough, or not behaving in a manner that you think is right. Guilt exists only in one's mind and is often out of sync with reality. It doesn't erase the past and can only hurt you by making you feel bad and draining your energy.

Negative self-talk and feelings of guilt are destructive and counterproductive. Are your intentions good, but your time and resources are limited? As a care partner, all you can do is your best with the skills and resources at your disposal. Acknowledge that you don't have all the answers, and reach out to others for help. No one is perfect. It is okay to make mistakes; we all do. Care partner guilt is almost unavoidable. You are going to feel guilty occasionally, but ask yourself what is triggering the guilt and give yourself permission to let it go. Accept that there will always be a gap between perfection and what you can actually do as a care partner.

As professionals, we encourage care partners to ask for help without having feelings of guilt. We have found in our many years of work that those who ask for help are stronger and more able than those who don't. Those who don't ask for help struggle with greater guilt because they feel inadequate to care for their loved one in the way they would like. They also burn out quicker, which can lead to sickness, fatigue, and unfortunately in too many cases, elder abuse. The end result of trying to do it all yourself is having less energy to offer your care partner.

Do Not Let Guilt Get the Best of You

- Determine what is causing the guilt.

- Try mentally and emotionally switching places with the person you feel you have wronged. How does he feel? Does he feel he was wronged? What does it feel like to be disappointed or ignored?

- You cannot change what happened, but you can make amends. If you can fix the problem that is creating this guilt, then do it. Learn from the situation, and move on.

- Reassess your expectations and make them more realistic. If you have tried all you can to change the situation that is causing the guilt, be kind and forgive yourself.

- Rely on something other than yourself for help. If you are spiritual, you can put your faith in your higher power. Friends, family, counselors, and others going through similar challenges are also good sources of support.

- Create a plan for the future, and approach it one step at a time.

- Forgive yourself. Everyone makes mistakes, and an important part of releasing guilt is forgiving.

Reducing Stress

Finding a way to let go of guilt is a necessary part of reducing stress. Stress prevents us from truly taking good care of ourselves and being the best care partners we can be. When we are stressed, our brains go into flight-fright-or-freeze responses. When we need them most, essential sections of our brains shut down. To make matters worse, when our bodies are in freeze mode, they store stress. The freeze response condenses stress in our bodies, preventing us from moving on after a stressful situation until we have released the stress that is lodged in our body.

Take a deep breath
Be kind and gentle to yourself
Expect imperfections
Believe in yourself

When something stressful happens or we begin worrying and thinking stressful thoughts, the amygdale in our brain tells our body to release stress hormones. It says, "I have so much to do. I will never get it all done!" The released adrenaline and cortisol flood our bodies, shutting down creative problem-solving parts of our brains. They also slow digestion and constrict blood vessels. The stress affects us physically, controlling how the body functions and how we think.

When we are under chronic stress, we do not have access to memories or problem-solving abilities. Stress is a liability that prevents us from being the best we can be. When we are able to relax, our brains can work at their full capacities. When we are relaxed, our bodies can heal themselves.

Accept Your Role

> *Claire had a very difficult lifelong relationship with her mother. She was quite resentful when her mom was diagnosed with Alzheimer's disease, and she wound up being the only person to actually care for her mother. She will tell you that she wasted years on her own anger and frustration at finding herself in charge of her mother's health and welfare. She had years of resentment and anger toward her, which only increased when she had to care for her.*
>
> *She thought,* Why me, poor me? What a cruel trick that has been played on me. *She kicked, screamed, argued, and nearly made herself sick with her anger and frustration. It wasn't until she couldn't stand it anymore that she sought the help she needed.*
>
> *For the first time in years, she was able to step outside her own unhappiness and observe the way others were with her mother. Claire could instantly see the difference in her mother once she was around others who found ways to make her smile and laugh and who didn't speak to her with condescension.*

"She was instantly happier and felt so much more secure—because she knew she was with people who were really engaged with her, who really liked her, sadly something with which I wasn't that familiar," Claire said. "What this brought about was a not-so-small miracle: the chance to have a completely different and much better relationship with my mother in her last two years than we'd ever had in our lives. We never did quite attain the mother-daughter connection I've seen so often with friends, with lots of hugs and 'I love you,' but we did learn how to relax around one another, even enjoyed our visits."

Claire spent her mother's last hours with her and says that even though her mother may not have known she was there, she knew. "And it made me feel human, like the daughter I'd always wanted to be," she said.

Make Peace with Your Feelings

It is very normal to be sad, angry, and even resentful. You might be sad because you miss the things this person used to do. You may be angry that you have to care for a person with whom you've always had difficulty getting along. You might get mad because of an unfair criticism or because too many little things went wrong throughout the day. Loss of control, lack of sleep, lack of free time, frustration, and disappointment can all make us angry.

Resentment is habitually felt toward the person being cared for when the care partner feels that his or her life is ruled by responsibility for a person who used to be an equal—but who now seems more like a burden. Resentment can also occur when care partners feel exploited because of real or imagined slights by other family members who they feel don't do enough to help. Feelings of sadness, anger, resentment, abandonment, or criticism can fester and evolve into anger and depression. This emotional stress can manifest itself in myriad physical problems, such as insomnia, digestive disorders, high blood pressure, heart attacks, heart disease, and headaches. Anger can explode and jeopardize relationships, and it can even harm others. Managing your anger and resentment helps your own well-being and makes you less likely to lash out at someone you care about.

These feelings of anger, resentment, and frustration are quite normal for care partners. If you are feeling these emotions, you are still a good person. However, non-verbally expressing these emotions to a person with dementia will only make your life more difficult. Seeking help to sort through these emotions is highly recommended. Resolving some of these emotions by talking with a professional or friend and accepting the diagnosis and moving forward can be very healthy. One way or another, these emotions will be expressed. It is best to do so verbally to someone who can help you sort out your emotions instead of taking it out on the person with dementia.

One family member described this struggle perfectly. "As the care partner, it is most important to recognize your own limitation to cope and give. Just because your family member needs you, you still have to respect your own feelings and not allow yourself to believe that you have to be a martyr. If feelings of resentment or fatigue or just being burned out start to surface, give yourself permission to have those feelings and take a break. We really only help our loved ones when we can be calm and loving. If you need to replenish yourself to get back to that place, let someone help or take over. It doesn't mean you are letting anyone down.

Don't let this disease consume you. You are still a person with a life and interests; try to maintain a balance. It is best for everyone."

Focus on the Present, Not on What Is Lost

The bottom line is that while it is hard to expedite the process of accepting your new role, it is necessary because you have a limited time to help your loved one as a care partner. Simply put, you must accept that your loved one has been given this diagnosis and make it your business to decide how you will live with it. We encourage you not to waste time being angry. Don't be depressed by what is lost; focus on what is still present.

Though this is easier said than done, the time you spend in denial will only make the person with dementia become more introverted and alone. Move forward by accepting this diagnosis and making the best of it. During this difficult time, it can be hard to think about anything other than what's going on, but try not to become so consumed by misery that you overshadow any glimmer of hope. Now that you have taken control of accepting what is happening, you can begin to design your schedule to include time to take care of yourself.

Make Time for Yourself

Beginning today, carve out some free time for yourself. Even if your loved one only requires minimum assistance right now, schedule some time to do something that is important to you. Try to schedule time once a week, at a minimum, though most people will need more. No one should have less.

Stay consistent for your sake, but more for the sake of your loved one with dementia.

Pick a day and time each week. Hire a companion or ask a friend or family member to stay with the person while you go out and do something on your own. Make sure that time is spent doing things that will refresh you. Many care partners feel guilty for leaving the person at home while they go out and visit with friends, attend a book group, or participate in a sport they enjoy. It is critical to realize that if you are not happy and healthy, you can never be an effective care partner. If you don't take breaks for your enjoyment, you will experience resentment, anger, and fatigue.

Simple Ways to Take Care of Yourself

- Tap into your higher power. Spiritual practice provides a sense of inner peace, a feeling of being centered and calm. Make time every day, even if it is only five or ten minutes, to pray, read spiritual passages, sing your favorite hymn, or participate in a religious ritual that is meaningful to you.
- Meet a friend for coffee.
- Take a weekly exercise class.
- Join a book group.
- Get a haircut or a manicure.
- Take a walk in the park.
- Play with your grandchildren.
- Check out some books or take a free class at the library.
- Go to the movies.
- Attend church.
- Write in a journal.

- Talk with someone in person, by phone, or through the Internet.
- Don't give up activities that are important to you.
- Eat nutritious meals.
- Get plenty of sleep.
- Participate in a sport you enjoy.

Think Positive Thoughts

Many people find that saying positive affirmations or mantras throughout the day helps reduce stress and fatigue. A mantra is a sound or words that are used to help create focus during meditation. Many people find repeating mantras to be a helpful stress-reduction technique, whether or not they meditate. Create your personal positive mantra or affirmation, and repeat it frequently.

Research has shown that positive thoughts and emotions change the neurochemicals in the brain that affect our mental, physical, and spiritual health. Saying an affirmation first thing in the morning starts you off in a positive mood and affects your decision-making for the day. If you forget to do this when you get out of bed, don't worry; mantras are helpful in stressful situations too. An affirmation could help prevent you from lashing out at someone and bring you back to a calm state. Some mantras that others have found effective include:

- This too shall pass.
- Tomorrow is another day.
- With God, all things are possible.
- I will accept the things I cannot change.
- I will look for the good in every day.

- Life does not have to be perfect to be wonderful.
- I have much to celebrate.
- I believe I can be kinder to myself.
- My pace is perfect.
- I am in control of my thoughts.

Where to Look for Help

Now that you know how you might spend your free time, it is time to find out what is available for your loved one to enjoy. Since this list is not comprehensive, always be on the lookout for new services being offered.

There is no extensive list of places to find great programs for people with dementia, but we have provided a list of resources and things to consider when evaluating your options. When you reach out to others for assistance, be as specific as possible about your needs. Describe the exact task with which you need help—whether it's driving your loved one out into the country to look at the fall leaves, taking him to a dentist appointment, staying with the person while you go out for an hour, or picking up some groceries.

Think about services you could barter. Could you trade time with someone who is also a care partner of someone with dementia? If a friend offers to sit with your spouse while you go grocery shopping, can you do his or her shopping at the same time? Can you say thank you with baked goods, a home-cooked dinner, or a handmade item, such as knitted socks or a pillow?

- **Office on Aging.** Call your local Office on Aging to see if there are any community programs available. Some might be subsidized by the state, others might have scholarships, and others might be private pay. Ask about all available programs for people with dementia, including any respite programs.

- **Eldercare Locator.** The United States Administration on Aging has a website that contains a variety of information on eldercare by topic. www.eldercare.gov

- **ARCH National Respite Network.** This website will help you locate respite services in your area (www.respitelocator.org).

- **The US Department of Health and Human Services.** The HHS offers a toll-free hotline for people in crisis. A nationwide team of crisis counseling experts has been set up to be available to help people who may be on the verge of suicide. People who are in emotional distress or suicidal can call at any time from anywhere in the nation to talk to trained workers who will listen to and assist callers in getting the mental health help they need. People will be provided with immediate access to local resources, referrals, and expertise (1-800-273-8255).

- **College Art Programs.** Start with local colleges that offer art therapy as a major. Second, look for schools that offer a therapeutic recreation degree. Contact the dean or the program director to ask if they have any mature students who would be interested in working individually with a person with cognitive impairment. If the student is meeting your loved one in your home, we recommend being present for the first few visits or until you are comfortable leaving them alone.

- **Music Schools.** Contact the school's dean or program director to see if they have any mature students who would be interested in working individually with a person with cognitive impairment. If the student is meeting your loved one in your home, we recommend being present for the first few visits or until you are comfortable leaving them alone.

- **Churches, Temples, and Other Houses of Worship.** Ask the pastor or rabbi if they know any members who might be interested in spending time with a person with dementia. There might be certain tasks that need to be accomplished in the house of worship that the person with dementia and someone from the congregation could work on together. These might include folding bulletins or straightening chairs.

- **The National Center on Caregiving.** The NCC works to advance the development of high-quality, cost-effective policies and programs for care partners in every state in the country. They have created a family caregiver network, a state-by-state, online guide to help families in all fifty states locate government, nonprofit, and private care partner support programs. The easy-to-use navigator lists programs for family care partners as well as resources for older or disabled adults living at home or in residential care communities (www.caregiver.org).

- **Home Care/Companion Agencies.** These agencies can usually be the most flexible to your schedule. See the appendix for a list of interview questions. They will be most helpful if you tell them the days and times at which you are looking.

- **Social/Medical Day Programs.** These will have set times during the day and might be available at least five days per week. See "Getting Your Ducks in a Row" for more information about these programs.

- **Geriatric Care Manager.** These people can help you to arrange any of these services in your area. They specialize in knowing what resources are available in your community and will help you make the necessary arrangements. In some cases, they will be available to spend time with your loved one while you take time for yourself. You can find a geriatric care manager in your area (http://www.caremanager.org/).

- **Veterans Administration.** If your loved one is a veteran, home health care coverage, financial support, nursing home care, and adult day care benefits may be available. Some Veterans Administration programs are free, and others require co-payments.

- **Fraternal Organizations.** Lions, Masons, Elks, Eagles, and Moose lodges, may offer some assistance if your loved one is a member.

- **Community Transportation Services.** Many of these are free for your care partner, while others may charge a nominal fee. Your local Agency on Aging can help you locate transportation to and from adult day care, senior centers, shopping malls, and physician appointments.

Fun Things for People with Dementia and Their Care Partners

- **Memory Cafés.** These casual social meeting venues are designed for those with progressive memory or cognitive impairment and their care partners, families, and friends. It is an opportunity to obtain information, resources, and fellowship. You can search online for a memory café in your area or go to www.memorycafes.org.uk or www.alzheimerscafe.com.

- **Artists for Alzheimer's.** This organization creates programs around the world for people with dementia that can be enjoyed by their care partners as well. Their website is regularly updated with new programs (www.artzalz.org).

- **Museum Programs.** Many museums offer specialized tours for people with dementia and their care partners. Look for them online by using the search term "museum and Alzheimer's disease programs."

All of these programs can radically change the way a person with dementia engages with other people and the environment around them. Care partners are often amazed to see their loved ones acting like their "old selves."

Take the time to do the research to find the programs and services available to you as a care partner and your loved one. With patience, you can tap into resources that can help your loved one remain busy and engaged in life—and you can enjoy his or her success!

Appendix

Health Care Summary for Emergency Personnel

The need to go to the emergency room is always a stressful situation. In order to be best prepared, create a folder with pertinent information and place it near your exit door. Make sure to keep this information updated after each visit to the physician.

Include a copy of the health care proxy, power of attorney, and insurance cards for the person with dementia.

Name: ______________________ Date of Birth: ____________

Medical History: ______________________________________

____

____

Current Medications:

Medication/Dosage	Start Date	Discontinued Date

Emergency Contact

Name Relationship

Address City, State, Zip Code

Home Phone Number Work Phone Number Mobile Phone Number

Preferred Hospital:

Known Allergies:

Conversations to Have With Your Physician

1. Explain past and current medical conditions and illnesses.
2. List all current prescriptions and over-the-counter medications (including over-the-counter supplements and medications like Benadryl or Tylenol).
3. Share with your physician if you think your loved one is depressed. Explain why you think this. Some reasons include losing a loved one, giving up driving, or retiring from work.
4. Report any changes in sleep patterns, including sleeping more during the day or waking up earlier in the morning.
5. Discuss changes in eating patterns, including overeating or under eating as well as eating spoiled foods. Also make sure to tell your physician if the person with dementia consumes alcohol and if so, how much daily.
6. Explain to the physician if the person with dementia has had any infections.
7. In many cases, your physician will:
   a. Collect urine for a urine analysis to rule out:
      - a urinary tract infection
      - dehydration
      - electrolyte disturbances

b. Draw blood for a baseline to check:
   - thyroid levels
   - anemia
   - untreated diabetes
   - kidney functioning
   - liver disease
   - vitamin deficiencies, including B12 and D

Long-Term Care Residence Checklist

Date and Time of Visit: __________ Contact Person: ________
Name of Long-Term Care Residence: ____________________
Address and Phone number: ____________________________

Many of these questions will help you to see how well a Long-Term Care Residence (LTC) is equipped to deal specifically with people with dementia. **Questions with an asterisk (*) relate specifically to dementia concerns.** In order to help you stay focused during your visit, look through this list of questions and highlight those that are most important to you.

Be sure those questions are thoroughly answered at each residence you visit.

Services

Do you have a specific unit for dementia care? *	☐ Yes	☐ No
If yes, can I see it?	☐ Yes	☐ No
Do you help residents with medications? *	☐ Yes	☐ No
Do you serve three meals a day?	☐ Yes	☐ No
Do you provide laundry service? *	☐ Yes	☐ No

Do you provide weekly housekeeping to residents' rooms?	☐ Yes	☐ No
Does your maintenance personnel provide free repairs or assistance if needed in the resident's room? *	☐ Yes	☐ No
Do you provide assistance to residents to get dressed and take a shower? *	☐ Yes	☐ No
Do you provide reminders to residents to use the bathroom? *	☐ Yes	☐ No
Do you provide assistance to residents who are incontinent? *	☐ Yes	☐ No
Are incontinent products included in the fee to live here?	☐ Yes	☐ No
Do you provide end-of-life care? *	☐ Yes	☐ No
Do you have a designated nurse for memory care?	☐ Yes	☐ No
If yes, how many hours a day?		
How do the residents contact the nurse? *		

____

____

Activities

Do you have a specific full-time activity director for the dementia unit?	☐ Yes	☐ No
Is the care partner staff also expected to do activities?	☐ Yes	☐ No

Given a potential resident's interests, do they have: *		
• ____________	☐ Yes	☐ No
• ____________	☐ Yes	☐ No
• ____________	☐ Yes	☐ No
• ____________	☐ Yes	☐ No
May I have a copy of today's activities? *		
What activities do most of your residents enjoy? *		
How many hours a day does your staff provide activities? *		

____

____

Staff

What is your total capacity for residents?		
How many residents are currently living here today? *		
How many staff members are working today? *		
How many staff members work at night? *		
What happens when residents get up at night? *		
Did staff say hello as I toured?	☐ Yes	☐ No
Did staff welcome me to this residence? *	☐ Yes	☐ No
Am I comfortable with the way staff interacted with residents?	☐ Yes	☐ No
Did staff talk to the residents instead of to each other? *	☐ Yes	☐ No

____

____

Residents

Speak with residents. What do they have to say about living there?	
How did the residents respond when I told them why I was there?	

____

____

Environment

Is the residence clean?	☐ Yes	☐ No
Is the kitchen floor smooth and not sticky?	☐ Yes	☐ No
Are the tables clean and not sticky?	☐ Yes	☐ No
Is the staff accessible in the same space as the residents (not away in an office)? *	☐ Yes	☐ No
Is the carpet in good repair? *	☐ Yes	☐ No
Are the walls painted, and are wall hangings secured? *	☐ Yes	☐ No
Are common spaces and hallways free of clutter? *	☐ Yes	☐ No
Is there a secure outdoor space that is easily accessible?	☐ Yes	☐ No

____

____

Logistics of the Move and Money

Do you do an assessment before a resident moves in? *	☐ Yes	☐ No
Do you visit a resident before he or she moves in?	☐ Yes	☐ No
Do you talk to a resident before he or she moves in?	☐ Yes	☐ No
Do you speak with a resident's physician or require paperwork from the physician?	☐ Yes	☐ No
What furniture is included? Can resident bring his or her own? *	☐ Yes	☐ No
Upon move in, which staff goes out of his or her way to spend time with the new resident? *	☐ Yes	☐ No
Are all services discussed above included for all residents?	☐ Yes	☐ No
If not, will you tell me before you bill me when another service is needed?	☐ Yes	☐ No
If I am not told in writing before I receive a bill, can I make the request to wait thirty days before billing begins?	☐ Yes	☐ No

____

____

Long-Term Care Insurance Company Questions

Name of Insurance Company: ______________________

Insurance Company Phone Number: ________________

Date Called: __________________________________

Name of Person You Spoke with: _________________

Policy Number: ________________________________

1. What services does my policy cover, and how much is the daily coverage? ____________________
2. Does my policy expire or run out? ______________
   a. If so, when? ____________________________
3. Does it cover in-home nursing? _________________
   a. If yes, what level of nursing care? ___________
4. Does it cover non-licensed home care workers? _____
   a. If yes, how much per day? _________________
5. Does it cover licensed home care workers? ________
   a. If yes, how much per day? _________________
6. Does it cover adult day programs? ______________
   a. If yes, how much per day? _________________
7. Does it cover respite programs? _______________
   a. If yes, how much per day? _________________
8. Does it cover assisted living? _________________
   a. If yes, how much per day? _________________
9. Does it cover nursing home? __________________
   a. If yes, how much per day? _________________

10. Is there a period of time I have to wait before the policy begins to cover services? ______________________________
    a. If so, how long? ______________________________
11. Are there any restrictions? ______________________________
12. Am I bound to a certain state? ______________________________
13. What do you require from me to activate my policy?

    ____
14. ______________________________?

    ____
15. ______________________________?

    ____

Blank Behavioral Log

Daily Log for (person with dementia): _____ Dates: ________
Behavior that is being documented: ____________________

	Check if Sleeping	If awake, write if person is engaged, agitated or has another behavior***
8:00 a.m.		
9:00 a.m.		
10:00 a.m.		
11:00 am		
12:00 p.m.		
1:00 p.m.		
2:00 p.m.		
3:00 p.m.		
4:00 p.m.		
5:00 p.m.		
6:00 p.m.		
7:00 p.m.		
8:00 p.m.		
9:00 p.m.		
10:00 p.m.		
11:00 p.m.		
12:00 a.m.		

1:00 a.m.		
2:00 a.m.		
3:00 a.m.		
4:00 a.m.		
5:00 a.m.		
6:00 a.m.		
7:00 a.m.		

***Bathroom, wanting to walk, doing art and crafts, physical therapy, dancing, singing, with group, cooking, eating, weeping, crying, fighting in care—document whatever behavior or activity the person is engaged in. *In order to best assess the changes in a person, objective, factual documentation is the best tool.* It is best to keep this log for a period of at least one week. This will give you a baseline. *At meal times, include if person eats all, half, or none of the meal.*

Quick Reading Check

Cover all but the first sentence with a piece of paper. Ask the person with dementia to read the first sentence aloud, and then gradually move the paper down the page and ask the person to read each sentence separately. Pay attention to any squinting, stammering, or stress that could indicate difficulty seeing the words. Ask the person which sentence is easiest to read. Use your observations and the person's response to determine the size of the reading material to provide. The first sentence is 16-point type, the next 24-point type, then 36-point, 48-point, and finally 72-point type.

The children are playing.

The dog is running.

The girl is pretty.

The water

is warm.

The sky

is blue.

Home Environment Safety Checklist

In and Out of Home

Can the person enter and exit the home independently?

Home Entry

Are there lights along the path of entry?
Are there lights at the door entry?
Are concrete and brick surfaces free from large cracks and uneven surfaces?
Are decks and landings stable and free from cracks, sagging, and exposed nail heads?
Are all banister rails easy to grasp, sturdy, and solidly anchored?
Do banister rails extend beyond the top and bottom steps?
Are gutter downspouts extended away from walks and driveway?
Are the paths free of shrubs, clutter, and debris?
Are there motion detector lights on the exterior?
Is there a ramp or non-step entry?
Does the garage door have an automatic opener?

Throughout the Home

Can person function and navigate throughout the home independently?

Lighting

Is lighting equally distributed?
Is there a light switch located at the entrance to each room?
Are light-sensitive night-lights used?
Are working flashlights kept by the bed?
Are outlets loaded appropriately, with no cube taps or daisy-chained extension cords?
Are all cords free of cracks and frays?
Are long cords kept off of walking areas?

Furniture

Is furniture arranged for a clear pathway?
Are all pieces of furniture sturdy and not easily tipped?
Can the person get in and out of chairs and beds easily?
Are chair armrests sturdy and easy to grasp?

Floor Surfaces

Are the floors free of piles?
Are all floors in good repair?
Are all linoleum surfaces secured to the floor?
Are all area and throw rugs secured to the floor with rubber backing or double-faced adhesive tape?
Does carpet pile height allow for easy movement throughout room?
Are the doorways free of any raised ridges?

Doors

Will doorways facilitate a wheelchair?
Are doorknobs easy to grasp?

Appliances

Are heating pads and electric blankets connected to timers?
Are the washer and dryer located on the main floor?
Is space available to move the washer and dryer to the main floor?
Can the person independently use the washer and dryer?
Are telephones located in each major room of the home (bedroom, living room, and kitchen)?
Do all fireplaces have spark screens?
Are smoke detectors and carbon monoxide detectors located on each level of the home, including the basement and near the bedroom?
Are smoke and carbon monoxide detector batteries checked at six-month intervals and changed annually?
Is there a medication management system in place and consistently used?

Bathroom(s)

Can the person get onto and off of the toilet independently?
Are grab rails installed by the toilet and tub?
Are non-skid strips or a mat used both inside and outside the tub?
Can the person safely get in and out of the shower/tub?

Kitchen

Is there a fire extinguisher located next to the stove?
Can the person prepare meals and dine independently?
Can the person move heavy or bulky objects in and around the kitchen?
Can the person use the stove independently?

Does the kitchen observe general safety guidelines while cooking?
Is the kitchen arranged so that food preparation and cleanup can be done from a chair?
Are all poisonous and flammable substances stored away from food products and the stove?

Stairs

Are all stair rails sturdy and anchored securely?
Do banister rails extend beyond top and bottom steps?
Are stairs free of slippery surfaces?

Interview Questions for a Potential Companion

Have you ever worked with someone who has cognitive impairment?
Preferably, you are looking for a companion who does have experience working with someone with dementia. Ask about any training courses completed.

If so, how would you describe your experience?
Some people will say they really liked it. That is a good answer. Others may say it was the same as caring for anyone else, which is still okay. If someone replies that it was really hard work but he or she liked it, you should consider that a less desirable response. Usually, that person will have had enough difficult experiences that he or she will begin to expect these negative outcomes and may not approach your situation with an open mind.

Tell me about a time you were flexible with one of your clients who had memory loss.
Listen to your instincts about which answer feels right. You are looking for someone who can give an example of a situation in which he or she made a change in their approach to communicating or providing care, rather than trying to change his or her client.

What do you think is the most important principle when care partnering with a person with this condition?
The answers can vary, but you don't want to hear anything about the companion changing the person with dementia - that would be a red flag. If the person talks about needing to take control of the person with dementia, that is not acceptable. If he or she talks about managing or controlling the *situation*, that is what you are looking for. That is all one can do. If you are unsure what he or she is expecting to do, be sure to ask - the difference is important!

How do you think you will spend your time during the day when the person with dementia is not in need of personal care?
Anything other than sitting and watching TV is the start to a good answer. Preferably, given the physical condition of your loved one, you want to hear the potential companion talk about going outside for a walk, playing games or reading together. Anything that shows he or she will engage your loved one is a good thing.

Are you willing to do activities if we help you to plan them?
You are looking for a person who will answer that he or she is willing, and preferably happy, to participate in activities with your loved one. He or she might be a little bit resistant because of uncertainty or their own lack of knowledge. If you sense any uncertainty, ask him or her why he or she is hesitating.

Are you comfortable sitting down and eating with the person with dementia?
In many settings, care partners are asked not to eat with the person with dementia. In some cases, the care partner

chooses to eat his or her own food or wants to eat at a different time. However, eating is a very social time, and a person with dementia benefits greatly, as does the care partner, by eating together. If the companion chooses to eat his or her own food, this is not a problem as long as this is acceptable to the person with dementia. In addition, a person with dementia often relies on what he or she sees other people doing to be a cue for what to do. If the care partner is sitting and eating with the person at the same time, this will serve as a cue, and help the person with dementia stay independent for a longer period of time.

Would you be interested in staying long term with us?
You would like them to say yes. Transition and change is very difficult for all of us and is even harder for a person with dementia. Your family and the person with dementia will have to welcome someone new into their life and begin to form a relationship of trust. If the care partner is replaced frequently, this will be hard for everyone and particularly unsettling for the person with dementia, as their coping and/or learning skills have become somewhat diminished.

Have you had a background check? Are you willing to have one?
Most licensed agencies will perform their own background checks, but it is still good to ask him or her. If you are hiring the care partner privately, it is good to do this just to be safe. Anyone who refuses to have this done is of concern. Ask him or her why he or she would prefer not to have a background check, and if he or she cannot give you a reason, we would suggest finding a different care partner.

Confirm their exact schedule.
It is good to have clear expectations of when the care partner is expected to work, for your sake and his/hers. If you are regularly changing the hours, the person might not be able to accommodate your needs. If he or she expects to have some scheduling issues (child care, car availability), it is good to know ahead of time. This way you can either put a plan in place to minimize these issues or interview for a second care partner who will be available in the event the first person is not.

Can you provide a list of references?
Recommendations from previous clients are very helpful. If they valued this person's work, the reference will often be very enthusiastic about the strengths of this person you are considering hiring. It is important to ask what the weaknesses of the potential companion are so that you know what to expect if, in fact, you do hire him or her. In addition, everyone's situation is different, and his or her weaknesses might not be something that is acceptable for your situation.

In general, this is an area where you want to be diligent. You need to be strong about references, ask the questions you need to ask, and not be afraid to offend the potential care partner. We are not suggesting being aggressive, but you do need to know if the person can furnish more than one reference. If not, ask questions and find out why. If this is the person's first job decide if you feel he or she will get along well with your loved one.

About the Authors

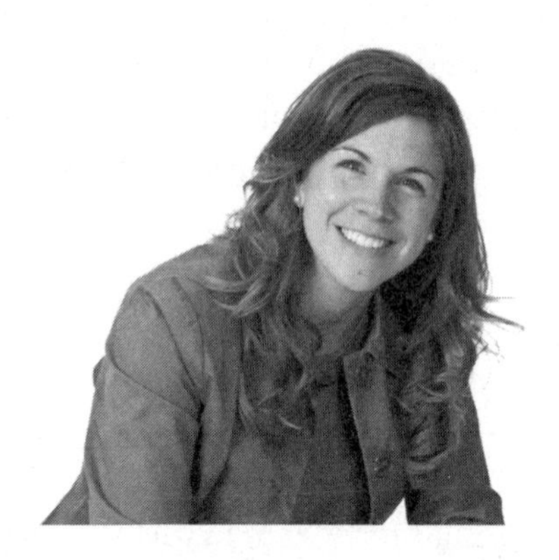

Kerry Mills, MPA, is an expert in best care practices for persons with dementia both in the home and in out-of-home health care residences and organizations. She is a consultant to numerous hospitals, assisted livings, hospice, home care agencies, senior day care centers, and nursing homes. In her twelve-year career in health care, she has served as executive director and regional manager for numerous long-term dementia facilities. She is an outspoken advocate for persons with dementia, lecturing in Hong Kong, Canada, China, Europe, and the United States.

Whether Kerry is participating in a symposium on health care at the United Nations, moderating a state-of-the-art Alzheimer's program at Boston's prestigious Coolidge Theatre, or simply meeting with a family, she exhibits a high level of enthusiasm and encouragement and delivers a message of hope regarding this debilitating disease.

Learn more at www.EngagingAlzheimers.com.

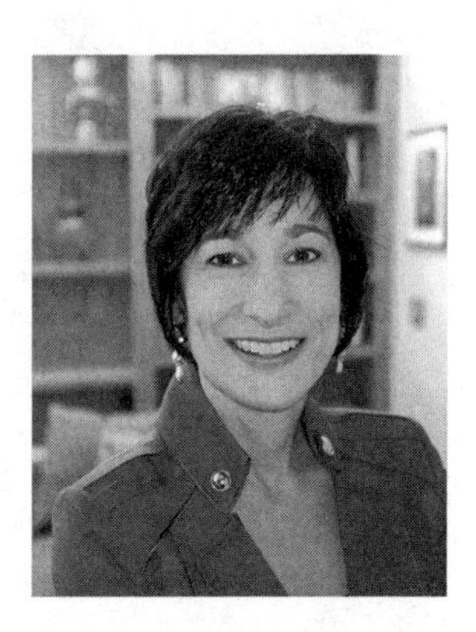

Jennifer A. Brush, MA, CCC/SLP has been working for more than twenty years to change the face of dementia care in hospitals, assisted living communities, nursing homes, and home care. She is a nationally recognized speech-language pathologist known for her work in the areas of memory and environmental interventions for people with dementia. She has served as the principal investigator on applied research grants that have examined issues pertaining to HIV/AIDS dementia, hearing impairment, dining, swallowing disorders, and the long-term care environment.

Jennifer offers interactive and educational presentations that help clients bridge the gap between current research findings and the care needs of people with dementia. Learn more at www.BrushDevelopment.com.